Date Due

Health Care Policy
in the
United States

Keith J. Mueller

Health Care Policy
in the
United States

University of Nebraska Press

Lincoln and London

© 1993 by the University of Nebraska Press
All rights reserved
Manufactured in the United States of America
The paper in this book meets
the minimum requirements of American National
Standard for Information Sciences –
Permanence of Paper for Printed Library Materials,
ANSI Z39.48–1984.
Library of Congress Cataloging-in-Publication Data
Mueller, Keith J., 1951–
Health care policy in the United States /
Keith J. Mueller. p. cm.
Includes bibliographical references and index.
ISBN 8032-3173-3 (cloth)
1. Medical policy – United States. 2. Medical
economics – Government policy –
United States. I. Title. [DNLM: 1. Health Policy –
United States. 2. Delivery of Health Care—United States.
WA 540 AA1 M895h 1993]
RA395.A3M84 1993 362.1'0973—dc20
DNLM/DLC for Library of Congress 93-15252 CIP

• • •

To the memory of Marie T. Mueller

Contents

Tables

Figures

• • •

Preface

As we approach the twenty-first century, the United States is at a crossroads in the development of health policy. During the 1980s the appropriate role of government in social policies was debated; newly elected national leaders argued in favor of reducing the level of the federal government's involvement in resolving social (human) problems. President Reagan was outspoken in his 1980 campaign and again in 1981: he wanted the level of federal social spending reduced and federal social programs trimmed. A variety of programs have been affected by these reductionist efforts. Health care programs are especially vulnerable because they represent the largest percentage of federal social spending, except for Social Security (projections are that Medicare will overtake Social Security in monies spent in the next ten years). An era of constraint in federal spending has brought reductions in the number of beneficiaries of some programs (such as Medicaid) and increased cost sharing by beneficiaries in others (such as Medicare). Government in the 1990s, however, seems once again to be focused on providing greater access to medical care by expanding eligibility in the Medicaid program and at least considering new programs to make health insurance available to those who are presently without that benefit.

This is certainly an appropriate time to ask what the commitments of government ought to be vis-à-vis the health care of its citizens. By the end of the 1980s, policy analysts and government officials realized that attempts to resolve any particular problem, such as high costs, would only exacerbate other problems, such as access to care for the uninsured. We now know that there is no magic bullet that will solve all the problems in delivering and financing health care in the United States. Those problems include: containing the ever-increasing level of expenditures devoted to health care, assuring access to care for the estimated thirty-three million to thirty-eight million uninsured Americans, meeting the health care needs of a growing elderly population, responding to the AIDS epidemic, and retaining a viable health care delivery system in rural America. The challenge confronting policymakers as we move toward the millennium is how to design policies that can successfully address one or more of these problems without exacerbating others or creating new ones.

•   •   •

The purpose of this book is to develop an analytical perspective on some of the major issues in health care delivery and finance. Theories developed by political scientists are used to help explain the evolution of health policy in the United States. They also provide a contextual understanding of how policies might be changed. Discussions of specific policies are presented as analyses of problems and potential solutions. We must move beyond a knowledge of political institutions and actors and into the realm of matching the best available science, which includes empirically based suggestions for reimbursement and other health care delivery policies, with the best available understanding of the pragmatic, or what is possible in the political arena.

Elected officials deliberating the future of health care policy are influenced by the political climate of the times (general ideological trends), the demands of an electorate, and the lobbying efforts of powerful interest groups. Specific policies are also products of detailed economic and social policy analysis provided to decision makers. Therefore, a thorough understanding of the development of health policy requires both knowledge of the actions of key actors within the political system and of the persuasiveness of research concerning specific policy suggestions. Our efforts to understand what might influence health policy in the next decade must be built on an explanation of how current policies were developed. Once we know how the expectations that built up in the political environment have been translated into policies we will also know what gaps remain. We should expect the policy debates of the next decade to focus on how to fill those gaps.

The first chapter of this book is devoted to a discussion of the politics of health care, including addressing why government would and does intervene in this arena and the expectations for intervention policies. Chapter 2 will build on this discussion by describing the current political environment and how policies are developed in that environment. Political forces that oppose further government action are contrasted with those that promote more proactive government policies. Chapter 3 will discuss problems that precipitate policies that determine levels and methods of payment in government programs. Chapter 4 will focus attention on specific policies to control expenditures in hospitals and for physician care. Chapter 5 will discuss a variety of policies designed to expand and assure access to and the availability of health care for all American citizens. Chapter 6 will review recent policies designed to improve the quality of health care. Chapter 7 will discuss the prospects for the reform of U.S. health care finance and organization in the context of other national systems. The final chapter will conclude with a discussion of the future of health care policy and the major policy initiatives we should expect to see.

This book represents a culmination of my thinking and writing about issues in health politics during the past seven years. I have been guided by the advice of several scholars who deserve special thanks here. John Comer has my gratitude for his patience in working with me as a coauthor of several analyses of health politics in state and local decision making and for his encouragement as I made the shift from studying general public administration to a focus on health issues. I owe a special debt to the Robert Wood Johnson Foundation and the faculty of the Johns Hopkins University for an enriching experience as a Robert Wood Johnson Foundation Faculty Fellow in Health Care Finance. In particular, I owe a great deal to Susan Horn for her valuable mentoring during that program and since. Finally, I want to acknowledge the support of two federal agencies who have awarded grants to projects I direct, enabling me to collect and analyze a wide variety of data: the Agency for Health Care Policy and Research and the Office of Rural Health Policy. Numerous other scholars have contributed to the thoughts expressed in this book, especially those active in the American Political Science Association and those who have offered suggestions in reviewing various drafts of this book. I thank them all. Of course, in the end, I am fully responsible for the content of this book.

On a more personal note, I want to thank my family, Gloria and Amy, for their emotional support and understanding during those unavoidable periods of frustration associated with a project of this scope. With them I share the joy of completion. A special debt is owed to my parents, Milton and Marie Mueller, for their understanding of the importance of nurturing the intellectual development of their sons.

1

. . .

The Politics of
Health Care

General support for government policies directed at health care delivery is found in the argument that access to health care is a right that should be guaranteed to all American citizens. There are two variations on this argument: (1) all citizens have a right to the same level of care, and (2) all citizens have a right to some minimum level of care. The American political system has chosen the second. The meaning of this choice cannot be found in any single policy but instead is implicit in the total of a number of narrowly written policies. In each instance, government has acted to provide access to medical care to narrowly defined groups, based either on economic need or special social circumstances. Benefits provided in government programs include those services necessary to treat life-threatening illnesses. Policies have been enacted to provide access to health care for specific groups otherwise unable to pay for and receive care—the elderly (Medicare), poor children (Medicaid), poor adults (Medicaid and local or state general assistance), the disabled (Medicaid and Medicare), veterans (Veterans' Administration), Native Americans (Indian Health Service), and patients in renal failure (Social Security benefits for kidney dialysis and transplants).

If we concede the argument that in our democratic society all individuals should be free to pursue their own concept of a productive life, providing a basic level of health care can be seen as a responsibility of government. What Norman Daniels (1985) has described as "normal species functioning" is necessary to realize the objectives in each individual's life plan. Specific health care services needed to enjoy other basic rights should be available to all; but this does not imply that all services, including cosmetic surgery, must be accessible by all people. As stated by Bayer et al. (1988, 583), "All Americans must have access to the full range of necessary health care services." The operative word here is *necessary;* government is not obliged to provide access to all the services citizens may desire or demand.

Significant debate exists over which health care services ought to be included in a basic tier, but the conclusion to the argument remains intact; there is a minimum level of services to which all citizens are entitled. The definitions of the level of services and the class of persons eligible for those services are often the result of political and economic debates as much as any predetermined right to care. Politically charged debates leading to expanded benefits include those in which victims of adverse health conditions, such as patients suffering from kidney failures or children waiting for organ transplants, present their cases directly to legislators. Economically motivated decisions are those that might restrict eligibility for benefits or the services rendered under new policies in order to minimize government spending. One of the most controversial applications of an economic criterion was a recent decision of the federal government to consider the costs for new procedures before determining whether or not Medicare will pay for them. A less pejorative use of economic analysis is to compare the cost effectiveness of competing medical treatments. That is, when a given condition can be treated in more than one manner, the costs of the alternatives can be compared—a form of cost effectiveness analysis.

The justification for having government pay some health care has a second supporting argument, that health care is a social good. That is, the benefits to the individual are also benefits to society. Policies related to public health, such as vaccination against contagious disease, are justified on these grounds. In order to secure the social benefits of the absence of disease, programs are established to promote preventive measures. For example, in 1988 the total cost to society resulting from all types of cancer measured in terms of lost productivity and health care expenditures was estimated to be approximately $65 billion (Office of Disease Prevention and Health Promotion 1988).

Regardless of the original justification used for government policies in this arena, specific mechanisms contained in policies and their subsequent adjustments are the products of actions taken by elected representatives. When the individual's ability to pay for care or the availability of health care providers fails to assure access for certain populations, government policies are enacted as attempts to fill the gaps. When access to services is assured, the government is justified in protecting consumers from harmful, inadequate, low-quality care.

Government action is predicated on the assumption that consumers typically lack the necessary information and expertise to assess the quality of care themselves (Marmor and Christianson 1982).

Although public policies influence the relationship between providers and patients, they do not control the specific content of what is done when providers and patients interact. Government programs have been established on the premise that groups of persons needed assistance in accessing quality medical care at a reasonable price, not that medical providers needed to be controlled by government. Therefore, the specific care management decisions of providers are not dictated directly by government, and those private decisions influence the quality and cost of care. The consequences resulting from the interaction of decisions made in the health care delivery system and the decisions made in the public policy system will determine the need for further governmental action.

Themes in Health Policy

Government policies have been enacted to resolve perceived deficiencies in health care delivery, defined in terms of quality of care, access to care, and the high cost of care. Although it is impossible to define clearly any given set of policies as accomplishing only one of these three themes, each has been emphasized in certain historical periods. Falcone and Hartwig (1991) have divided the twentieth century into four policy periods: quality during 1900–1960, access during 1961–72, cost containment during 1973–80, and decrementalism since 1980. The fourth period they describe is actually a blending of the three earlier themes, under the guise of decentralizing decisions from the federal government to the states and reducing overall public spending. Responses to any particular thematic concern are driven by political needs to relieve pressure generated by specific interests in society: medical professionals (defining and protecting quality), consumers (demanding easier access), or payers, who include taxpayers (demanding lower expenditures). In current debates concerning health policy issues, the results of health services research and policy analysis demonstrate the interrelatedness of the three themes, and policies are designed based on the results of that research and analysis.

QUALITY

Policy activity in the early years of the twentieth century focused on the development of the health professions and methods of delivering health care. Even before then, in 1869 the Commonwealth of Massachusetts created a state board

3

of health. By the early years of the twentieth century, state governments were established as the regulators of health professionals, determining the qualifications necessary for licenses to practice. State governments also regulate health care facilities, requiring them to meet specific conditions in order to be certified. New York took the first step in 1894 by requiring health standards for private facilities certified by the State Board of Charíties (Levine 1984).

Government concern for the quality of care became more obvious as the practice of medicine became more "scientific." In the early 1900s attention turned to the curriculum being used in medical schools to prepare physicians. The National Confederation of State Medical Examining and Licensing Boards recommended a uniform curriculum to all schools in 1904 (Litman and Robins 1991). Major reforms in medical education were suggested in the 1910 Flexner report, which encouraged a university hospital–based model for education. Following that report, both the medical profession and government continued to promote scientific education as the proper preparation for physicians (Starr 1982a).

Scientific methods were also applied to developing medications. The first Food and Drug Act was passed in 1906. Biomedical research began to receive government support in the first half of the twentieth century, with the National Cancer Act of 1937 and the Public Health Service Act of 1944. The medical community's emphasis on the scientific approach to treatment helped increase the importance of hospital-based care. The transformation of hospitals into centers of medical excellence (rather than almshouses) began after the Civil War but saw its principal manifestation in the early 1900s (Starr 1982a). Since hospitals became the source of high quality medical care, the federal government undertook another quality-based initiative in 1946 when it enacted the Hill-Burton legislation to provide grants for the construction and expansion of hospitals.

Government policies promoting better care can be interpreted either as protecting consumers or as supporting health care providers. The former interpretation is based on government's propensity to promote the general welfare of the citizenry by influencing those services that directly affect the personal welfare of citizens. The U.S. government has done so with other social welfare policies, including child labor laws, safety and building codes, food programs, and direct assistance. In each instance, the government's involvement comes only after policymakers believe the private sector cannot or will not take the necessary actions. In the case of the early health care policies just discussed, the private sector could not be expected to police itself without the power to enforce certain standards concerning providers (the state licensing laws), and resources were not sufficient in the private sector to promote the rapid development of the scientific approach to medicine (hence Hill-Burton, the grants for scientific research, and the support of medical education to promote the use of knowledge gained through scientific research).

A second interpretation of the policy initiatives of the early twentieth century is that they were promoted by the health care professions to support their centralized control of the permissible practices in health care delivery (Starr 1982a; Feldstein 1984). Providers are expected to defend quality care as they define it, to the exclusion of alternative providers and styles of care. For example, physicians emphasize the "medical model" for treating patients rather than a biosocial model that emphasizes the roles of other professionals.

ACCESS

The theme of expanding access to care began developing at the same time as the policies designed to promote greater quality of care in the delivery system. In fact, the Hill-Burton legislation can also be interpreted as legislation intended to promote access to care because it financed the construction of many hospitals in rural America where none had existed before.[1] The legislation also required hospitals to provide "charity care" as a condition of receiving funds, but not necessarily to all those who otherwise had no access. Other policies related to hospitals were even more obviously enacted with expanded access in mind. State and local governments in the early twentieth century supported hospitals that provided care to the poor in their communities (Stevens 1982). The practice of publicly supported community hospitals became increasingly common during the 1940s and 1950s.

The theme of access to care was obvious in early suggestions for a system of national health insurance (NHI), including those offered by President Truman in the 1940s. Partly as the result of a massive campaign launched by the American Medical Association (AMA), Truman's proposals were not enacted, but the seeds were planted for his advisors and others to harvest over a decade later. In the interim between advocacy by some for NHI in the 1940s and the federal government's entry into financing benefits in the mid-1960s, private insurance schemes provided access to health care for an increasing number of Americans.

1. The interpretation of the Hill-Burton program is still weighted to quality because the emphasis was placing a certain delivery style (hospital based) in every American community.

5

This was an important development in American health policy—an approach to health care finance that relied on private parties, not government, to develop and implement plans to spread the burden for payment so that each individual could afford access to care. Private health insurance began with a modest plan at Baylor University Hospital in 1929, but the concept gained in popularity as part of labor-management agreements in the late 1940s. The development of private health insurance schemes was encouraged by exemption from wages that counted toward limits during World War II and by creating tax deductions for health care insurance premiums (Munts 1967). In 1948, 2.7 million workers were covered by insurance; by 1954 that number grew to 12 million workers and 17 million dependents. By the end of that year, more than 60 percent of the total U.S. population had some form of insurance (Starr 1982b). These insurance policies answered most of the health care finance needs of the American middle class and with some exceptions they continue to do so. This pattern of responsiveness to the needs of that large (and politically influential) segment of the American population helps explain the difficulty of achieving a broad program in the United States for government-sponsored health insurance.

In the 1960s, the U.S. government devoted more attention to problems of access to care. The growth in private insurance coverage was not providing complete coverage to all groups in society. In particular, the elderly and the poor faced catastrophic expenses not covered by health insurance. As the decade began, national health insurance was seen by many as the best means of assuring access, but a shift occurred to focusing instead on the needs of particular groups. As early as the Truman administration and definitely by 1958, congressional attention turned to the health care needs of the elderly (Marmor 1973). In 1960 Congress enacted legislation, the Kerr-Mills program (Public Law 86-778), which provided federal grants to state government programs of assistance to the elderly. That program, though, did not guarantee comprehensive coverage of all medical expenses incurred. Considerable latitude was given to the states, and only four states provided the full range of benefits permitted in the program (Marmor 1973). By the time of the Lyndon Johnson presidency, momentum built for legislation to protect the elderly from the financial catastrophe caused by health care expenditures.

Even with the momentum, however, the incremental nature of American politics prevailed. Rather than a radical departure from existing mechanisms of financing health care, Congress created an insurance plan, supported by public dollars, in which the elderly shared the cost of care through monthly premiums

6

for physician services and copayments for hospital services. Even this incremental measure became possible only after a landslide election of Democrats in 1964 and the bargaining that obtained the support of Congressman Wilbur Mills (chair, House Committee on Ways and Means) (Marmor 1973). Medicare, and its companion program Medicaid (care for the poor was added to Medicare in part to compromise with a physician-drafted proposal), established the precedent that government should facilitate access to health care among those unable to secure it themselves.

Other programs enacted to expand access have included the National Health Service Corps and legislation supporting rural health clinics to expand geographic access, student assistance programs to expand the pool of health care workers, legislation to expand a system of emergency medical services, and health clinics for inner cities to extend medical care services to those underserved areas. The health planning legislation of 1974, although enacted at the beginning of the cost containment era, can be seen as a last gasp to continue the theme of expanding access. The program was intended to contribute to continued efforts to enact NHI by forcing rational planning on the system in preparation for more extensive federal financing (Mueller 1988a). Although efforts to expand access did not receive much emphasis from 1974 until the early 1990s, the theme was nonetheless continued, through appropriations for the health worker programs and continuation of Medicare and Medicaid.

COST CONTAINMENT

The third theme of federal policy, cost containment, reached domination in the late 1970s. Legislation was enacted to contain rapid increases in health care expenditures. The Health Planning Act of 1974 was a major effort in this battle designed to reign in costs by preventing unnecessary expansion in the health care delivery system. Through application of Certificate-of-Need programs, states were to constrain the expansion of hospitals in particular; the theory was that each new hospital bed increased overall expenditures, regardless of the rational need for that bed. As a program to contain health care expenditures, health planning was a failure (at least in the judgment of many in Congress). Efforts to contain cost increases continued with price freezes during the Nixon administration and with suggestions to control hospital prices followed by a voluntary restraint during the Carter administration, and they culminated in the program of prospective payment for hospitals enacted in 1983.

Along the way, other reforms in the health care delivery system were encour-

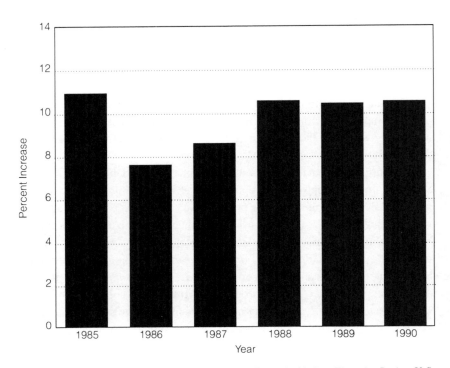

Figure 1.1 Increases in health expenditures, 1985–1990. From *Health Care Financing Review,* U.S. Office of National Health Statistics, Washington, D.C., 1985–90.

aged by federal programs. The most notable of these was the promotion of health maintenance organizations (HMOs) during the mid-1970s. HMOs are believed by many to promote a more efficient form of practicing medicine. Evidence is overwhelming that HMOs achieve savings by realizing lower rates of hospitalization among their patients than would otherwise be expected. State governments have contributed to efforts to introduce reforms into the system by permitting the creation of preferred provider organizations (PPOs). These schemes constrain costs by encouraging consumers to seek care from the least costly physicians and hospitals in their communities.

In spite of all the policies enacted in recent years, health care costs increase every year. In 1989 alone, total health expenditures jumped 10.4 percent. Figure 1.1 displays annual increase in health care expenditures in the second half of the 1980s. Public officials face the grim realities of what those figures mean every year when budgets are prepared. For the federal government, health spend-

8

ing now represents 14.8 percent of the budget, and Medicaid expenditures represent as much as 20 percent of state budgets.

For the average citizen the cost of care is obvious when the costs of childbirth are reviewed. In 1989 the average total cost for delivery was $4,334 and for cesarean sections $7,186. Physicians' fees alone were $1,639. The costs may not seem high to women with private insurance that pays their costs, but 17 percent of women do not have health insurance, and another 330,000 have private insurance that does not include maternity coverage (Minor 1989). For government the cost of maternity care is of direct concern as it affects the Medicaid program, which spent $1.2 billion in maternity care in 1985. Questions of how to use advanced technology are also associated with delivery, since neonatal intensive care units, by keeping premature babies alive regardless of their prospects for a healthy life, drive expenditures ever upward. In addition, expenditures for childbirth have increased because of a higher percentage of deliveries being completed as cesarean sections.

Since cost containment remains a dominant theme in health care policy, the specific policies implementing that theme will be discussed in much greater detail in the balance of this book. Since health care expenditures have continued to escalate even after many efforts since 1974 to control them, policymakers remain anxious to adopt other measures to stem the tide. Of special concern are the costs of technologies that continue to be introduced into the system and the costs of caring for an aging population.

THE THEMES COMBINED

Although cost containment continues to receive attention in policy discussions, access to care has again emerged as a major concern. As of 1991 there are at least thirty-one million and as many as thirty-eight million Americans without any form of health insurance. Evidence from surveys conducted by the Robert Wood Johnson Foundation indicates that the uninsured experience reduced access to services, either because they seek care less often or they are turned away by providers when they do seek care. Legislation has been discussed by states and the federal government to relieve the problems of this population group, with programs enacted in Massachusetts, Oregon, and Hawaii to accomplish that objective. In addition to those without any health insurance, those whose insurance is not comprehensive and for whom premiums and copayments are increasing can also be viewed as subject to financial problems when they try to obtain health care. The elderly are another major group that may experience financial problems accessing care. Prescription medications and long-term care are not included as benefits in the Medicare program. Congressional concern for this access problem was obvious when it enacted the 1988 Medicare Catastrophic Coverage Act. Although that legislation went down in the flames started by lobbyists for the elderly in 1989, the concern for access remains.

Geographical access has also become a major policy issue again. The Rural Health Coalition in the House and the Rural Health Caucus in the Senate have both been active in promoting legislation to help sustain existing services and bring more health care services to rural communities. Their efforts have focused on keeping rural hospitals viable, and their most dramatic achievement was passing legislation in 1989 to equalize Medicare payments for rural and urban hospitals.

The details of the measures to expand access will be discussed more fully in the balance of this book as a major theme of current health policy. Cost containment and access form two pillars of current policy efforts. The third historic theme of health care policy, concern for quality, is also experiencing a renaissance. Several specific policy initiatives are indications of this renewed concern. First, funding to evaluate new treatment methods and diagnostic tools is increasing. Second, funding for outcomes research has increased, focused on the question of appropriateness of medical procedures. Evidence has shown that practice styles (how to treat specified conditions) vary widely, even within the same geographic region and certainly across regions. Third, the quality theme is evident in the activities of regulatory bodies such as state licensing agencies, facilities inspectors, and federal regulatory agencies (particularly the Food and Drug Administration). Fourth, the Omnibus Budget Reconciliation Act of 1987 included provisions to improve the quality of care in the nation's nursing homes.

In summary, the two principal thematic pillars of current policy efforts are cost containment and access to health care. Concerns for quality of care remain, especially related to efforts to improve cost effectiveness in the delivery of health care. In enacting policies consistent with these themes, American governments (national and the states) begin with the assumption that the current system of financing and delivering health care is basically sound and that policies are needed to improve that system. Therefore, policies are incremental in nature and shy away from NHI. This book will conclude with a discussion of the possibility that the traditional approach to health policy is ineffective and that as a result we may see a break with tradition in the next decade.

Various groups in society are suggesting policies that would incorporate all current payment schemes into a single scheme of national health insurance. A group of physicians has joined this growing sentiment, along with some major corporations and several special commissions (Stevens 1989). Cost containment is still the driving force behind such recommendations, but access to care for the uninsured is a major problem also addressed in current policy suggestions. The array of special efforts to contain costs, especially those that try to reduce unnecessary services, has contributed to the debate about the balance between cost containment and quality of care provided. The three principal themes driving health policy in this century are all emerging at the same time, which may precipitate a different approach to federal policy. A convergence of pressures from major interest groups, including some physicians, may drive policymakers to consider radical changes in our approach to health policy in the United States.

Congress and others interested in reforming the current system of financing health care with an eye toward cost containment and expanding access are increasingly turning to health services researchers and policy analysts for specific suggestions. Congress took a major step in this direction in 1989 when it created the Agency for Health Care Policy and Research (incorporating what had been the National Center for Health Services Research) and appropriated millions of dollars to support research that would examine the effectiveness of a variety of medical procedures. The two major cost containment policies of recent years—prospective payment for hospitals and resource-based payment for physicians—have been ideas implemented by creating special commissions to review research and analysis before recommending specific rates of payment. These efforts are encouraging in that high quality analysis is being used to develop public policies, but a great challenge remains—using the best research that can be produced to shape analysis that shapes policies designed to achieve a combination of objectives simultaneously.

The Changing System of Health Care Delivery

An important contributing force to the reconsideration of public health policies originates in changes in the system of health care delivery in the United States. As the system for delivering medicine seems increasingly driven by profit motives, the tendency to impose constraints on that system may grow. As economic considerations force consolidation within the delivery system, concern will grow about access for those who lose traditional sources of care. New relationships between health care professionals and their employers in group practices and other health care organizations may make physicians willing to consider new schemes for delivering care, since they have already sacrificed some of their professional autonomy for the good of the organizations in which they work.[2]

In 1982, Paul Starr (1982a) broke new ground in writing about the health care delivery system when he suggested that medicine would be practiced by corporations, not individual professionals. Starr's predictions have not yet proved to be entirely true, but the trend toward corporatism remains intact (the specific numbers will be presented in chapter 3 when this subject is considered in greater detail). The classic economic model of medical care being delivered by suppliers to those demanding the care seems more appropriate than the traditional Hippocratic oath model of the physician serving all those in need of care regardless of ability to pay or other characteristics. The supply of care is affected by the desire to earn a profit, or in the case of nonprofit organizations, to generate funds for reinvestment; hospitals are closing that cannot receive sufficient revenues, other hospitals are declining to serve those unable to pay,[3] and physicians limit the number of patients they will see who are not insured by a private carrier. Those demanding the care are also forcing changes in the system. No longer are all prospective patients merely reporting symptoms to physicians and then placing complete trust in the physicians to diagnose and provide treatment. Instead, in part because of pressure from private insurers, patients are now initially more selective about when to seek medical care and whom to see for the care. Also, insurers are making providers accept predetermined fees for specific services. All of these changes in the health care delivery system make it increasingly possible to take the next radical step and allow for greater government intrusion; the previously sacrosanct patient-doctor relationship has already been altered.

2. The historical basis for physicians' opposition to government programs has been that those programs would interfere with the doctor-patient relationship. That argument loses its strength, however, when that relationship is not controlled exclusively by a physician paid directly by the patient. Salaried physicians are already following guidelines set by their employers. With other schemes such as preferred provider agreements and utilization review gaining in popularity, physicians are much less in control of their practice environments. Therefore, one of their major objections to government programs is weakened considerably.

3. This is accomplished primarily through not offering those services used by the uninsured, particularly emergency care (the emergency care capacity is limited). There have been, however, documented cases of outright refusal to treat those without insurance.

The use of a wider array of delivery mechanisms in the health care system opens new possibilities for health policy to achieve objectives of access and cost containment. As discussed earlier, government already began such initiatives with respect to HMOs in the 1970s. Now policies can take advantage of the increasing use of outpatient procedures to replace hospitalization (the prospective payment system used in Medicare does this at least indirectly by basing payment on shorter hospital stays), the use of paraprofessionals to perform procedures formerly done only by physicians (rural health clinics take advantage of this change), and increased competition among health care providers (preferred provider arrangements do this).

The new economic environment in health care delivery also presents some problems for policymakers. When corporate interests control health care delivery there is a distinct risk that they will go out of business, leaving access problems behind. This prospect is apparent in the corporate involvement in HMOs around the country, particularly after one large firm, Maxicare, declared bankruptcy in 1988. Corporations active in buying hospitals are also subject to economic failure. Short of economic failure, problems are created for public policy when for-profit medical providers begin to reduce costs by limiting access to services. Some of them, such as Humana Women's Hospital in Tampa Bay, Florida, specialize in treating only those patients able to afford programs giving special treatment (including champagne with meals after delivery). Questions of the moral right to care arise in these circumstances, and those questions are likely to become more common.

A final implication of changes in health care delivery deserves mention in this introductory chapter. Advances in medical technology continue to challenge our abilities to finance all possible care for all citizens. Major technological advances continue to be made in diagnostic techniques. As the last vestiges of the health planning program die (Certificate-of-Need laws are being repealed or liberalized), we can expect increasing competitive pressures for more widespread ownership of diagnostic equipment and affiliation with medical teams conducting highly sophisticated procedures. These activities produce a great deal of revenue for corporate institutions and medical care practitioners, and the proliferation of those activities is another consequence of changes in the delivery system. Government policies may very well have to include some form of rationing if society determines that the continued proliferation of every new technology is unaffordable. The state of Oregon has already confronted this issue in the context of its state-run Medicaid program, deciding that spending more money for prenatal care and other services is preferable to spending Medicaid dollars for certain organ transplants.

The relationship between the health care delivery system and government policies will become increasingly important in the next decade. Each clearly affects the other, and government decision makers will need to understand the nature of that interaction as new policies are developed.

The Political System

Government activities in health policy are important to all those concerned with how medicine is practiced and financed. In 1987, government payments for health care services totaled $207.3 billion, 41 percent of all revenues for health care providers (Levit and Freeland 1988). Government payments are a major source of income for key groups of providers; Medicare payments alone may account for more than 50 percent of the revenues of many hospitals. Government payment is now linked to the financial survival of some health care institutions, and it influences the level of payments from other sources who follow the lead of government in determining rates of payment for particular services. Therefore, it is crucial to understand how and why government policies change.

Specific policies will be determined by actors operating in political institutions, influenced by variables affecting their political judgments including economic conditions, advances in technology, and analyses of policy alternatives. Changes in health policies should follow changes in the institutions and/or changes in the political culture. This working hypothesis has obvious applications to the shift during the years 1977–81 from federal policies emphasizing regulation to policies promoting competition in health care delivery. Federal decision makers responded to economic analyses that discounted the effects of regulation and promoted competition and to changes in the political atmosphere that brought Republicans to power in the Senate and increased their numbers in health committees in the House.

The legislative environment for health policies has changed in recent years. There are many more trained staffers in Congress involved in shaping health policies. There is a greater general interest in health policies that affect such a great share of the federal budget each year. In both federal and state governments there is a much greater concern about the budgetary impacts of policy decisions.

Congress has a greater institutional capacity than was true in earlier decades to deal with the complexities of health policy. Congressional staffs are often augmented by expertise available through programs such as the Robert Wood Johnson Foundation Fellowships in Health Policy, congressional fellows, and other professional fellowship programs. The executive branch also benefits from a number of such programs, including the White House Fellows Program. The expansion of staff capabilities has improved the ability of Congress to respond to changes in the economic environment and to analyze existing policies. This in turn enables more rapid shifts in policy direction when there are shifts in legislative focus, such as the 1981 shift in partisan control of the U.S. Senate. The cadre of health analysts in legislative offices also increases incentives to create legislative solutions to problems in health care delivery, because the measure of success of many of the analysts is their ability to influence policy.

Economic analyses receive greater attention than they had previously because the expanded staffs are able to understand the methods as well as the findings. The analysis is partisan analysis, however, consistent with what Lindblom (1965) has described. For each partisan position, economists and other analysts can supply the ammunition to defend or oppose a particular economic solution to problems such as physician reimbursement. The tasks of decision makers (and their staffs) are to sift through discipline-based rhetoric (such as political science, economics, planning) and pronouncements of the best solutions to find the most desirable policies, given their own political judgments.

Differences of opinion concerning approaches in public policy are thrashed out in the political arena. Given the propensity of a democratic political system to compromise whenever possible, policies are often enacted that disappoint professional analysts and may not be able to succeed as well as intended. Even incremental changes in policies, however, can accumulate and become dramatic shifts (Lindblom 1979; Mueller 1984).

Summary

Considerations of health policy in the United States must be cognizant of changes in both the political arena and the health care delivery system. The interactions between those two are the grist for the health policy mill. Questions of how the health sector behaves have dominated policy debates in recent years. Inducing competition has been the policy preference, and private for-profit firms have increased their share of the health care delivery system. Pressures in the political system to control public budgets dominated the debates in the 1980s and will continue to do so in the 1990s.

This decade will also witness increased attention to the problems of those excluded from access to health care for financial reasons, which will strain the policy system's ability to meet both health policy objectives and the general objectives of budget control. Therefore, even more attention will be devoted to how policy actions interact with patterns of delivery and finance in the private sector to assure access for all. The current debates bubbling up in Washington, D.C., from corporations, physicians, and others about the possibility of a system of NHI are an indication of this focus. Current demonstration programs financed by the federal government for Medicare and Medicaid beneficiaries to increase their use of HMOs are also signs of this emerging direction in policy.

The direction of health policy will depend as much on changes in the political system as on changes in the health care delivery system. The climate within which politicians enact policies can and often does influence the specifics of those policies. Hard facts such as the plight of the thirty-three million to thirty-eight million uninsured Americans do influence the directions of policies. In addition, the analysis of research results helps shape the specifics of public policies, as has been the case for hospital and physician reimbursement policies in the Medicare program. The specific contents of policies, however, will still represent the product of partisan debate, albeit informed partisan debate.

2

. . .

The U.S. Political System and
Health Policy

Health policies in the United States are the products of deliberations within a
political system. Although objective considerations of problems and potential
solutions may inform policymakers, their ultimate decisions will nevertheless
reflect political ideology at least as much as rational problem solving. In that
context, what are the possibilities for new policies designed to treat major problems in health care delivery? What variables will influence the nature of the policies? What are the forces that may bring change in policies? These questions
can be answered by reviewing approaches used by political scientists to explain
the operation of American government institutions and applying those descriptions to health care policy.

The most common explanation of policy activity is one based on the role of
interest groups and the incremental policies that result from compromises designed to satisfy their demands. The political system is expected to treat all
group demands equally and promulgate policies that steer a middle course intended to create the least disturbance among the various groups. That approach
is successful as long as the middle course is apparent and addresses the problems being considered. Such an obvious course of action is becoming increasingly difficult to find, as more complex problems fail to yield to simple solutions.

The importance of interest group pressures may diminish as complex problems prove less and less amenable to simple incremental solutions that do not
displease any of the groups. As problems have become more complex, the political system has evolved by adding professional staff to both the legislative
and the executive branches of government and by specialization among the

elected officials. These changes can lead to different and less influential roles for interest groups and others accustomed to wielding dominant influence in previous years. In short, the stage may be set for more radical change in policies.

This chapter includes a discussion of the traditional description of the American political process. The interaction of interest groups and elected officials is emphasized, as is the natural resistance to radical change in public policies. The changes in the political system that have occurred in the 1980s are then described, and their effects on the traditional understanding of American politics is analyzed. Finally, prospects for new directions in health policy, given the evolution of the American political system, will be discussed. Illustrations drawn from considerations of health policy will be used throughout the discussions.

The Traditional Description

American politics has been characterized by the pursuit of collective interests by various groups in society. In the resulting pluralist environment decisions are the result of various groups competing for a share of society's resources. In that competition the strong—that is, the largest and wealthiest groups—prevail. The preferences of those groups are to protect their advantages. Innovative, nonincremental policies are resisted by the established groups because such measures undermine the bargaining practices designed to reduce threats to any established interests. The stability of the system is assured because most groups are satisfied with the benefits they receive, even though the result for any single group is less than optimal. Interest-group pluralism affects health policy just as it does any other policy debate in American politics. There are powerful interest groups involved in health care politics who resist any major change (Alford 1975). These interest groups include physicians, hospitals, medical schools, insurance companies, and government agencies. They seek to maintain their respective controls over those aspects of health policy of most concern to them. Collectively, they have resisted significant change in the system, such as suggestions for national health insurance.

Alliances are formed among dominant interest groups and members of the legislative body to protect and enhance the interests of those receiving benefits from government programs. Commonly referred to as either iron triangles or subgovernments, these alliances combine members of legislative committees, executive branch agencies, and interest groups. Each member of the alliance receives benefits from current programs. The legislators are able to demonstrate to their constituencies economic benefits from government spending in their districts; agencies are able to expand their programs; and interest groups are direct recipients of services through government programs. An illustration of this is the alliance between researchers, the National Institutes of Health, and the health subcommittees of appropriations committees. The concept of subgovernments is particularly useful in explaining how programs are constantly expanded and never radically changed—locking in continued benefits for the current set of actors.

A somewhat different legislative strategy can be exercised by especially powerful interest groups who seek to prevent government from enacting policies inimical to their self-interests. These groups use political muscle, through campaign contributions and the ability to convince large blocks of voters to follow their lead, to persuade legislators to support their position. These groups are likely to concentrate their efforts on important legislative committees, often opposing new programs or dramatic expansion of existing programs. This is especially true of groups such as the American Medical Association (AMA), which traditionally oppose any prospect of government intrusion into what they view as their sphere of influence (specifically, in the case of the AMA, the doctor-patient relationship). When change occurs, these groups will do all they can to make it as favorable to their self-interests as possible, even if that means reducing the chances of achieving the program's objectives. For example, the AMA opposed national health insurance in the 1940s and 1950s, and Medicare in the early 1960s. Once it became obvious, however, that a program of health care coverage for the elderly would be enacted, the AMA used its lobbying powers to be certain that the program did very little to change the mechanics of physician reimbursement and did nothing to interfere with the doctor-patient relationship.

There are instances when interest groups are advocates of significant change in public policy. The American Association of Retired Persons (AARP), for example, advocates a major new program to finance long-term care for the elderly. During the 1950s and 1960s, organized labor advocated national health insurance (NHI) and is doing so again in the 1990s. The natural inclination of the political system, however, is to change slowly. Combined with the opposition of powerful interest groups this natural inertia is very difficult to overcome.

Identifying the important interest groups, the sources of their influence, and their objectives helps us understand policy development. Paul Feldstein has identified seven principal health associations: AMA, American Dental Association, American Nurses' Association, American Hospital Association (AHA), Blue Cross Association, Association of American Medical Colleges, and American Association of Dental Schools. Since his writing, the Federation of Health Care Systems (for-profit institutions) should be added to the list. Feldstein found that these groups behaved in manners consistent with group interests, especially in striving to guarantee professional autonomy and improve income:

> Health professionals are also interested in their autonomy and in controlling their own working conditions; however, autonomy and control are likely to be correlated with higher incomes in that the professionals who have the highest incomes are also those who have the greatest autonomy and control over their activities. What seems to be an issue of autonomy is really one of income. A simple income objective should be sufficiently accurate to be used by itself. (Feldstein 1977, 11)

He further describes five types of policies favored by those groups that: increase demand for their services, enable firms to be reimbursed for services as price discriminating monopolists, lower prices of complementary inputs, increase prices of substitutes for their services, and restrict additions to supply. In short, the professional groups are seeking to retain their dominant position in the health care delivery system.

Other groups are active in lobbying efforts related to particular policies. The AARP is certainly a strong advocate for expanded health benefits for retirees. Unions and business groups are concerned that government programs minimize costs (taxes) to their members. The interests of these various groups at times clash. The analytical question is: which group has the strength to prevail?

Certainly the size of the group matters, but how the size is seen by the politicians is more important than mere numbers. How a group is concentrated in a representative's district and/or state is important (is it a large percentage of eligible voters? of campaign contributors?). How the group is concentrated in its own industry is also important (Salamon and Seigfried 1977). Both size and concentration are measures of the resources the group uses in the political process. Size can be measured in terms of money the group has available to contribute to political campaigns and/or the number of members who can be mobilized in an election. Persuasive lobbying is also a valuable resource, although normally it cannot overcome money and votes. In the 1990s policymakers are increasingly looking for suggestions based on research results and policy analysis. The persuasive power of interest groups is increased when their arguments respond to that need. The days of simply taking a position based on authority, as was once the tactic of the AMA, will no longer suffice.

The groups with the most resources are not always victorious; they may be resisting inevitable changes in public policy. Such was the case for provider groups who fought against Medicare; they changed their strategies in the face of obvious defeat. The scenario is repeated periodically when change is inevitable (as happened in the late 1970s and early 1980s concerning hospital payment under Medicare). Interest groups normally at a disadvantage in resources can be most successful when acute problems require new policies that conflict with the desires of more powerful groups.

AN EMPIRICAL EXAMINATION OF THE POWER OF GROUPS

There are two principal strategies appropriate to examine the influence of interest groups in developing public policies. First, the evolution of a particular policy can reveal the importance of various factors in shaping the policy, including the roles of various interest groups. This approach will be taken in subsequent chapters as particular policies are examined. Second, aggregate votes in the U.S. House, Senate, and state legislatures can be analyzed using measures of interest group strength as independent variables, controlling for other potential influences. Findings using that approach are presented here.

Political science literature is rich with efforts to explain roll-call votes. A set of core variables has proved to be most successful as independent factors in statistical tests: party identification, liberal/conservative ideology, region (especially for Democrats), and nature of constituency (particularly safe vs. competitive districts) (see Fiorini 1974 for a thorough review of this literature). Despite the strong statistical power of party identification and ideology as explanations of votes, considerable variance in voting remains unexplained. Other constituency characteristics are likely to explain that variance. This is especially true of votes on issues that do not necessarily challenge party loyalties. No single dimension of a member of Congress's profile, such as party identification, should be expected to carry equal significance in explaining a variety of policy votes. Clausen (1975) is most persuasive in raising this argument, finding different explanatory models for different policy dimensions in congressional voting between 1953 and 1964.

Interest group lobbying efforts play a role in defining issues and influencing votes in Congress. Smith sees congressional decisionmaking as a two-stage process involving the interpretation of relationships between issues and career goals, and the task of groups is to persuade members that the votes they desire contribute to career goals (Smith 1984). The groups with the most resources valued by representatives of Congress should enjoy the most success. This hypothesis was tested for health issues voting by Feldstein and Melnick (1984) in an analysis of votes on HR 2626 to control hospital costs (favored by President Carter in 1979). They found contributions of the AMA to congressional campaigns to be of little importance in explaining votes after the effects of three other variables were considered: political party, the annual percentage increase in hospital expenditures in a state from 1977 to 1978, and the percentage of the state's population on Medicaid. Using higher hospital cost increases as an indicator of hospital opposition to the legislation, they concluded that the hospital expenditure variable was the most explanatory. The pattern they uncovered was what Smith and Clausen alluded to in their work: issue-specific forces will influence congressional voting when career objectives (reelection) are not obviously at risk. Members of Congress were more influenced by party affiliation than by the interests of state governments. They also evidenced a general reluctance to change (the hospitals agreed to a voluntary price restraint before the final vote).

The vote on hospital cost containment did not reverse any expectations that Congress would protect the interests of established health care providers. Several other votes in recent years, however, have not been in the best interests of providers. These have included supporting HMOs, requiring health planning and Certificate-of-Need (CON), establishing professional standards review organizations (PSROs), and enacting cost containment legislation. In each instance, legislation resulted from compromises that eased at least somewhat the concerns of medical professionals. Nonetheless, the legislation was in principle contrary to the best interests of the professionals. These votes, which number nine when several votes on certain issues (such as HMOs and health planning) are included, are treated below as a set of dependent variables for further analysis of the power of certain independent variables specific to health care in determining the outcomes. The votes recorded during roll call are treated as the dependent variable; absences are excluded and paired absentee votes are included.

An analysis of these votes in the House of Representatives employed the fol-

22

lowing independent variables in Probit[1] models: conservative voting record[2] of the member of Congress, party identification, contributions by 1972 health political action committees, state medical association (MA) membership (as a percent of nonfederal physicians), and state/local share of Medicaid expenditures (Mueller 1986). The model was successful in accounting for over 80 percent of the variance in all nine votes, and as much as 92 percent in two votes (one HMO vote and the PSRO vote). Ideology was consistently significant in explaining outcomes. Conservatives predictably opposed policies that increased the involvement of government in financing and encouraging changes in health care delivery. Nearly as significant as an independent indicator of votes was the membership in the state medical association (MA). In only two votes (HMO votes in 1975 and 1978) was the MA membership not a statistically significant explanation of the likelihood of a member of Congress voting against increased federal involvement in health care finance and delivery. The MA measure tapped a critical resource, electoral support through voting power. The voting power of the MA included both members and patients. Further, the professional assessment of legislation by physicians from the home district may influence a representative's thinking on health-related issues.

The constituency dimension of the MA lobby was more important during the 1970s than were monetary resources. The 1972 health PAC contributions were not important in explaining votes, but it should be kept in mind that this particular measure is not a sophisticated measure of contributions. The measure of 1972 PAC contributions was imprecise and that may account for its weak performance in the statistical model (Cantor 1982).

The measure of state/local contributions to the Medicaid program performed well as an explanatory variable, being independently significant in explanations of these votes: 1972 health planning, 1975 health planning, and 1975 HMO. It approached significance in equations explaining the 1978 health planning and 1973 HMO votes. In all cases it predicted votes in favor of expanded federal government activities.

1. Probit is a statistical technique that permits analysis of the independent effects of independent variables on a dichotomous dependent variable (such as a yes or no vote). The effects are measured as probabilities of a yes vote, given an above- or below-average measure of the independent variable.

2. The conservative voting record of a member of Congress is a composite score reported by the Conservative Coalition, based on several votes during a congressional term.

The importance of the two variables indigenous to health policy (medical association interests and state government interests) varied according to the technical aspects of legislation. For example, the MA variable was consistently important, except for the last HMO votes. The major battles concerning HMOs were waged in 1973, after which the physicians felt victory was theirs because the original HMO legislation included multiple requirements that made future success difficult at best. Interestingly, the measure of successful physician lobbying shifted from MA membership in the 1970s to PAC contributions (measured in 1982) in the 1980s (Mueller 1986). The Medicaid contribution variable was most significant when the issue was clearly one of cost containment. This was obvious in the 1975 HMO legislation, which would have weakened the requirements that HMOs provide comprehensive care. Such a move would have lessened their impact on the overall costs of care in the community, hence keeping Medicaid costs high. The Medicaid variable also showed strong support for health planning, which was another way of containing costs by preventing unnecessary capital expansion.[3]

An analysis of U.S. Senate votes during the 1970s showed similar results to the House analysis just described (Mueller 1985). In this analysis thirteen votes were included: six concerning HMOs, three concerning health planning, two concerning hospital cost containment, one concerning manpower, and one concerning Hill-Burton funding. The thirteen votes were combined into a single index and regression procedures were used to test the explanatory power of the following independent variables: state/local Medicaid share, the number of proprietary hospitals in the state as a percentage of all hospitals, state MA membership, and political party. The measure of political party in this research was divided into Northern Democrats, Republicans, and Southern Democrats, enabling the single variable to measure both party identification and ideology.

The findings for the Senate votes varied a little from the House findings. The measure of proprietary hospitals was significant, indicating some promise in using this industry measure as a means of testing for the influence of hospitals. Hospitals consistently opposed the reform legislation used in this analysis. Consistently associated with passage of the legislation, although not quite at a .05 level of significance, was the measure of state/local contribution to Medicaid expenses. The MA membership variable was also associated with opposition to the policies but at weaker levels of significance.

3. As discussed in chapter 1, the evidence concerning health planning has persuaded many that it has not lowered health care expenditures, but in the early and mid-1970s the hope was alive that the program would have that effect.

What can we say about the development of health policy in Congress given these findings from an analysis of House and Senate votes? Since ideology is the principal explanatory variable we cannot expect too many individual representatives to change their voting patterns over time. They will change their votes, however, if the issue is redefined, as was the case in the different HMO votes. If their ideology is applied differently (from a primary concern of protecting the status quo to a primary concern of saving government funds, perhaps), their voting pattern may change. We can expect some changes in votes because of an issue not having a clearly defined ideological content. This would give the interest groups involved in lobbying a greater opportunity to interpret the issue for members of Congress. The importance of state MA membership in several votes supports this conclusion. When the issue confronting Congress is principally a technical issue to modify the health care delivery system we should expect those groups most directly affected (either positively or negatively) to be influential in determining the outcome of the legislative process. Their influence may be felt in committee deliberations as indicated in the case study literature, and/or in the floor votes, as the roll-call analysis has indicated.

Interest group activity occurs in the context of the specific political environment surrounding particular arguments. Thus, there was a difference in the effects of AMA lobbying between 1946 and 1964 (NHI debates and Medicare). The political environment seems to dictate the nature of the debates among interest groups. When Congress became concerned about health care expenditures in the mid- to late 1970s, provider groups had to fight harder to defeat legislation inimical to their interests. They increased the intensity of lobbying efforts—and the size of contributions to political campaign funds. When they did, their influence on voting (as in the health-cost containment vote) became more obvious.

INERTIA IN THE FEDERAL SYSTEM

State governments are directly responsible for many health programs, including immunization, environmental health, and public health. They also influence decisions concerning health care delivery through licensing professionals, providing professional education, regulating health care institutions, financing health care delivery (especially through the state-run Medicaid programs), providing the rules of the game for court actions (particularly malpractice litigation), permitting alternative delivery systems (requiring enabling legislation and approval), and establishing and operating certificate-of-need (CON) programs.

Interest-group politics are apparent in state policy development, and provider groups have a vested interest in any policies that affect their abilities to control their own practices. Lee and Estes (1983) found that organized health professionals were active in every state and involved in shaping health policy in nearly all. They found that policy differences across states reflected the demands of health care professionals. Daniels and Regens (1981–82) found support and lobbying strength of a state's medical association, along with the birth rate of the state, to be more important in explaining physician-assistant licensing than measures of wealth, industrialization, and innovativeness in the states. Brown (1983) found medical lobbies to be influential in designing CON statutes. Health providers were influential in determining the composition of health systems agencies (Checkoway 1981) and state policies toward the aged (Estes 1979). Barrileaux and Miller (1988) found that physician supply was an influential variable in explaining differences in state expenditures for Medicaid. When the interests of health professionals are somehow at stake in a given state policy, we should expect them to exert as much influence as possible.

As was true in national politics, provider influence in policy development in the states is associated with resistance to change (opposing HMO licensing, health planning initiatives, and CON statutes). Some changes, however, would be favored by providers if their interests are promoted. The best example of this would be changing statutes related to malpractice to make it more difficult to win large awards in judicial proceedings.

Traditional descriptions of the policy process, based on the theory that interest groups compete with one another for benefits from the political system, predict very little change from current policies. Policies develop a momentum of their own, protected by those groups deriving benefits from them. Change can occur if new groups gain sufficient power to override the interests of the entrenched groups, but such a change in political strength is unlikely. Change can also occur if the positions of the groups change, also unlikely. Providers dominate the policy debates, giving them the power to resist policy changes likely to diminish their control over their own income and practice authorities. The political system is based on compromises among interest groups and incremental policy change, facilitating domination by provider groups.

Changes in the Description

As Brown (1988) argues, policies have been developed to please simultaneously a variety of interest groups (providers, consumers, payers) because it has been possible to spend whatever resources are necessary, layering new programs onto old. The ineffectiveness of efforts to contain prices or to rationalize the system of health care delivery has been tolerable because of expanding resources. For the past few years, however, resources have not expanded dramatically. The constraints on the system have caused many to question existing policies and the propensity to satisfy new demands through program expansion. In this atmosphere, ideas and analyses are receiving as much attention, if not more, than the desires of particular interest groups.

Three modifications of the traditional understanding of American politics are most appropriate to explain the activities in health politics in recent years. First, the number and type of active participants in health policy discussions have expanded beyond the once-dominant provider interest groups. Second, policymakers have become more concerned with the technical dimensions of problems, reflecting the changing nature of the issues they confront. Third, the institutions of American government have undergone subtle but important changes that have served to lessen the dominance of particular interest groups in public policymaking. The three modifications will be discussed in the following pages by using the concepts of issue networks, the politics of ideas, and policy entrepreneurship, respectively.

ISSUE NETWORKS

Interactions among staff, legislators, and various interest groups form issue networks important in the development of legislative initiatives. This is a broader pool of actors than the traditional subgovernments. Any actors who participate in the process of developing particular policies are included (Heclo 1978). Heclo defines a network as "a shared-knowledge group having to do with some aspect (or, as defined by the network, some problem) of public policy" (103). Participants in the network share common knowledge and are aware of each other's perceptions of issues. The network is fluid—different groups come and go. Heclo uses a health-policy illustration to make the argument:

> At any given time only part of a network may be active and through time the various connections may intensify or fade among the policy intermediaries and the executive and congressional bureaucracies. For example, there is no single health policy network but various sets of people knowledgeable and concerned about cost-control mechanisms, insurance techniques, nutritional programs, prepaid plans, and so on. At one time, those expert in designing a nationwide insurance system may seem to be

27

operating in relative isolation, until it becomes clear that previous efforts to control costs have already created precedents that have to be accommodated in any new system, or that the issue of federal funding for abortions has laid land mines in the path of any workable plan. (104)

Actors within these networks relate to each other based on shared policy concerns, often irrespective of other labels such as party identification. Debates and discussions are couched in terms of the policy under consideration: "Like experienced party politicians of earlier times, policy politicians in the knowledge networks may not agree; but they understand each other's way of looking at the world and arguing about policy choices" (Heclo 1978, 117). A careful reading of the comments included in the Pepper Commission Report by the various elected officials on that commission underscore this point.[4] For example, Senator Durenberger voted against the commission's recommendations but said, "There was a strong consensus that the national social insurance system must be both overhauled and used to supplement individual resources—especially for low-income people—for basic health services and for long-term care." He added: "The final success is that we agreed in principle to move toward more uniform national standards for health benefits and for access to social insurance protection" (Pepper Commission Report 1990, 182). Another dissenter, Representative Bill Gradison, said simply: "We share the same goals but differ on how to reach them" (Pepper Commission Report 1990, 193). The issue network is rallying around the drive to move toward a different system of social insurance.

The issue network model is distinguished from traditional notions of iron triangles because a given network is not dominated by a few groups and because it will change as different actors assume more active roles depending on the precise nature of the discussion. Decision makers will be influenced by what they perceive to be the relevant constraints and opportunities in their policy environment. Ripley suggests these principal elements of the policy environment: (1) perceptions of decision makers of trends and events salient to them, (2) perceptions of need for a specified action, (3) perceptions regarding the potential impact of various options for action and the techniques needed to implement them, (4) the perceived history of government attention to a problem, and (5) the established patterns of attitudes relating to the issue area (Ripley 1972). The

4. The Pepper Commission was a special congressional commission charged with recommending policies to broaden participation in health insurance.

policy-relevant environment is defined in part by the actions of policy-makers, but events and general social trends may precipitate changes in the environment regardless of activities of decision makers. In health care, improvements in surgical techniques and the effectiveness of drugs led to a growing demand for organ transplants, which changed the policy environment during the 1980s, facilitating federal legislative initiatives to fund a national organ-sharing network.

The degree to which advocacy groups can push their perceptions of events and trends will help shape the policy-relevant environment. Groups must concentrate on interpreting events and issues to convince members of committees that specific actions are required (or not required). Testimony during public hearings can be understood in this context, just as Smith (1984) has used this framework to discuss lobbying tactics more generally.

Much of the activity within the policy-relevant environment takes place in particular committees in Congress: the House subcommittees on Labor, Health and Human Services, and Education (Appropriations), Health and Environment (Energy and Commerce), and Health (Ways and Means); and Senate committees on Labor and Human Resources, Finance (Health subcommittee), and Appropriations (Labor, HHS, and Education subcommittee). Issue networks form around the activities of these committees: Medicare financing issues addressed by the Senate Finance and House Ways and Means committees, suggestions for health care spending by the Appropriations committees, and new programmatic initiatives by the House Subcommittee on Health and the Environment and by the Senate Committee on Labor and Human Resources.

Some groups, those commonly mentioned in discussions of subgovernments, are consistent participants in most issue networks concerning health policy. These include the AMA; AHA; Federation of Health Care Systems (formerly Federation of American Hospitals); major insurance companies (Blue Cross and Health Insurance Association of America, HIAA); Department of Health and Human Services (DHHS, formerly Department of Health, Education, and Welfare, HEW); members of the committees and their staffs (particularly the subcommittee and committee majority and minority staffs); and business interests, through the Washington Business Group on Health (WBGH).

Other groups and individuals become important for certain issues. Professional groups with interest in particular programs, such as the American Association of Health Planning, will participate as active members of the network when those issues are debated. Academic researchers and consultants will be participants when their particular expertise is needed to analyze policy suggestions, such as discussions of hospital payment.

Iron triangles, or subgovernments, imply a fixed relationship among groups, agency staff, and elected officials that does not change over time and resists changes in policies. Issue networks imply a much more fluid relationship among a broader array of actors. Change in policy is facilitated when the influence within the network shifts. For example, strong pressures from the senior citizens lobby (primarily the AARP) to expand health care benefits for Medicare recipients, combined with analytical findings concerning the burden of payment imposed by extended and/or repeated treatments in a given year, can lead to new policies to change Medicare cost-sharing schemes. The fluidity of positions in the issue network was obvious in actions of various groups vis-à-vis the Medicare Catastrophic Coverage Act of 1988. That legislation resulted in part from lobbying efforts by the elderly through such organizations as the American Association of Retired Persons (AARP) to receive expanded Medicare benefits, including assistance in meeting expenditures for physicians and hospital care. Others in the issue network, including members of Congress and their staffs and members of the Reagan administration, worked to change legislation satisfying the needs of the elderly while still meeting government objectives of not adding to the budget deficit. The end product was celebrated by all as a major expansion of the program, until the AARP and others turned against it. Groups representing the elderly returned to old-fashioned politics and viewed the program as contradictory to their position that Medicare programs be provided without additional cost to the elderly. Their opposition, combined with a successful grassroots campaign, motivated Congress to repeal the legislation one year after it was enacted. Some provisions were retained or added to other legislation, such as requiring states to provide Medicaid benefits to all pregnant women and infants in families with incomes below federal poverty guidelines, mammography benefits for women in the Medicare program, and the protection of spousal income when the other spouse enters a nursing home.

New actors may enter the networks when policy shifts occur. The increased importance of budget officers resulted from health expenditures increasing rapidly and becoming a target for budget cuts to meet deficit targets (as has been the case in recent federal budget cycles). There are no iron triangles in issue networks, only a variety of groups and individuals among whom degrees of influence may change, dependent upon the nature of the issue being discussed and the dominant ideology of the time.

POLITICS OF IDEAS

Closely linked to the notion of evolving issue networks is the concept of a politics of ideas. Ideas are based on the climate of opinion—conceived broadly as the general public opinion or more narrowly as the collective opinion of policymakers. Kingdon (1988) writes of the former in describing ideas that "sweep across the land," fostering changes in policy. The power of particular ideas may bring policy changes despite the assumed power of interest groups normally expected to oppose specific suggestions (Derthick and Quirk 1985), or when general economic conditions would indicate different choices (Kelman 1987, Quirk 1988).

The power of ideas is in many instances a persuasive explanation when others seem to fail. Quirk (1988) argues strongly that this is the case when examining deregulation as a policy change in the late 1970s and early 1980s. The explanations offered by the economic perspective, he argues, are incomplete and cannot account for instances of policy change that are inconsistent with the demands placed on the political system by powerful interest groups.

Any particular idea may fester for a considerable length of time in the issue network before gathering steam and becoming the dominant idea of the time. Potential incubators of ideas include the community of scholars and other professionals analyzing particular problems (Mueller 1988b). New ideas, especially early in their lives, are often resisted by members of the "subgovernments" (Heclo 1978, 105), but networks of issue experts can also provide the analysis advocates need to overcome that resistance (Derthick and Quirk 1985). Creating a system of national health insurance was an idea included in early discussions of social security during the Franklin Roosevelt administration. Strong opposition of the AMA helped keep this idea from being included in the social security provisions recommended by the Roosevelt administration and subsequently enacted (Morone 1990a). Nevertheless, members of the issue network, especially Wilbur Cohen and his colleagues, continued to work on the details of a program addressing at least the health insurance needs of the elderly. In 1965 a constellation of circumstances facilitated action on this idea: a landslide Democratic party electoral victory, a commitment of support by Chairman Mills of the House Ways and Means Committee, a growing number of elderly poor, pressures on state budgets resulting from service provision to the elderly poor, and an increasing political strength among the elderly. Action happened quickly once the window was open, so the years of analytical and political work were essential in preparing to move quickly on that opportunity.

31

Particular ideas are especially likely to emerge in a context of a general change in policy direction. In health care politics the shift in emphasis to cost containment provided a favorable environment to consider regulatory policies and health planning legislation in the 1970s. A later shift in general government policies toward deregulation encouraged new approaches to cost containment; as a result, prospective payment was an idea whose time had come, despite previous opposition from such traditional groups as the AMA and AHA. No particular interest groups strongly advocated prospective payment; it was the idea generated by analysts (beginning with federally sponsored research in the late 1970s) that gained favor in a Congress looking for some means of controlling expenditure increases.

Ideas for significant changes in policy direction, such as prospective payment according to a fixed schedule, may require years to evolve from an analytical suggestion to concrete policy. The final steps in becoming policy will be a function of opportunities created by a legislative environment in which decision makers are willing, even anxious, to consider radical new directions (Kingdon 1984).

POLICY ENTREPRENEURS

Once members of the issue network become the purveyors of new ideas in the political environment, a further impetus for legislative change comes from actors within the legislative body who champion the change. These legislators are policy entrepreneurs who are linking career advancement to their ability to secure enactment of major policy initiatives.

Traditionally, policy leadership is located in the offices of subcommittee (or committee) chairpersons of the relevant authorizing committees. There have been three principal sources of such entrepreneurship in the development of health care legislation—the Senate Committee on Labor and Human Resources, the House Energy and Commerce Subcommittee, and the House Ways and Means Health Subcommittee. Influential individuals have chaired those committees in recent years: Senator Kennedy (with an interruption by Senator Hatch from 1981 to 1986 when the Republicans were the majority party), Representative Paul Rogers (until his retirement in 1978), Representative Henry Waxman (since Rogers's retirement), Representative Dan Rostenkowski, and Representative Fortney "Pete" Stark (the latter two chairing the Ways and Means Subcommittee).

In discussing the careers of entrepreneurs in Congress, Jones and Woll (1979) identify the careers of Representative Rogers and Senator Kennedy as

32

being built around their reputations as health policy experts. Rogers developed a strategy of building his career in Congress by developing numerous initiatives in health care policy even though the issue was of minimal concern to his Palm Beach, Florida, constituents. He saw this policy as one on which he could have an impact because others in the late 1960s and early 1970s were not addressing it:

> Among his colleagues in the House he was recognized as the leading figure in health policy on the Hill, Mr. Health of Congress. Over a three-year period Rogers was directly responsible for such legislation as the Health Research and Health Services Act, the Health Information and Disease Prevention Act, the Health Revenue Sharing and Nurse Training Act, the Developmentally Disabled Assistance Act, the Comprehensive Alcohol Abuse and Alcoholism Prevention Treatment and Rehabilitation Act, the National Foreign Flu and Immunization Program, the Safe Drinking Water Act, the Health Professions Education Act, the Clean Air Act, the Rural Clinic Service Act, the Medicare and Medicaid Antifraud and Abuse Act, the Arthritis, Diabetes, and Digestive Diseases Act, the Emergency Medical Services Act, the Indian Health Care Improvement Act, and the Health Maintenance Organization Act. (Jones and Woll 1979, 45–46)

Rogers successfully became the center of a network that included his and committee staffs, the biomedical community, administrative officials, and the research community. Rogers's successor to the Energy and Commerce Subcommittee, Henry Waxman, has also become a "Mr. Health" in Congress. He has successfully retained subcommittee jurisdiction over major health care legislation, so the process identified by Jones and Woll of legislating through amendments to previous legislation has continued under his leadership.

The counterpart to the House version of Mr. Health continues to be the Senate's Edward Kennedy. His early aggressive strategy of gaining jurisdiction over a wide variety of health programs continues: "By 1972 Kennedy was the Mr. Health of the Senate. As soon as he gained the chairmanship of the Health Subcommittee, he increased its activities geometrically from what they had been in prior years" (Jones and Woll 1979, 62).

Policy entrepreneurs emerge from sources other than subcommittee chairs. Various members of Congress may choose to champion particular causes either because of a special interest in a particular issue, as part of a strategy to gain visibility, or a combination of both. Forums outside the traditional authorizing committees for these entrepreneurs include investigative subcommittees, special committees (for example, the Select Committees on Aging), and ad hoc groups in Congress (for example, the Senate Rural Health Caucus). The number of such outlets has grown in recent years and the number of congressional staff assigned either directly or indirectly (through the various committees and subcommittees) to individual members has also increased dramatically (Smith 1988). Not only are the members entrepreneurs, individual staff are also entrepreneurs, seeking to establish their separate careers as specialists of value not only to Congress but also to better paying private employers (Malbin 1980). Those staff include persons responsible for health issues in every office. Some are there as health policy fellows, sponsored by various foundations. Those individuals in particular are anxious to have some influence on the development of health policy legislation and will work to develop policy initiatives their employers can sponsor in Congress.

A combination of entrepreneurial staff with a policy-oriented member is often the genesis of legislative initiative. As Congress decentralized in 1973, the opportunities for policy entrepreneurship increased: "The practical problem is that Congress's fractionalized workload results partly from recent procedural reforms that strengthen the subcommittees and partly from the advantages that entrepreneurial staffs bring to chairpersons and other members who seek to gain credit for new policy initiatives" (Malbin 1980, 244). Especially in the House, networks of persons involved in policy issues develop and communications within those networks become sources of legislative development (Fox and Hammond 1977).

Issue networks serve as incubators of change. The length of time from suggesting change to the final enactment of new policy initiatives will vary depending upon the political climate of the times and the sophistication of analysis supporting specific suggestions. The latter can be addressed by advocates of change within the networks before the political climate is ripe for change. The role of policy analysts, for example, can be to strengthen the analytical support for policy suggestions and translate the analysis into language easily understood by those expected to make the policy changes. The suggestions can be constructed in a manner that is politically persuasive, even if that means moving away from analytical purity (Mueller 1988b).

Changes in the political climate occur as problems are redefined or as new problems not previously addressed arise. These scenarios create opportunities for change if there are specific suggestions ready for policy enactment and if there are political actors who will champion the change. Policy entrepreneurs, then, take up the demand for change that had been developed by others in the issue network and carry it forward.

Others may become entrepreneurs by working through legislatures. Wilbur Cohen did so from a vantage point outside the legislature in working for Medicare in the 1960s as an official in the president's administration. Members of interest groups can become initiators, particularly on the details of legislation. The American Health Planning Association, for example, worked closely with congressional staff in developing the 1974 Health Planning Act. On occasion, individuals outside the legislative body can exert direct influence in legislation. Health services researchers played a key role in developing legislation to establish a medical effectiveness initiative to conduct research designed to improve the quality of medical care. Although ideas may come from any actor in the issue network, introduction of specific legislation incorporating the suggestion will be a task assumed by the policy entrepreneur in the legislative body.

Modifications have been suggested in the traditional interest-group approach to describing policy development in order to incorporate more recent research literature about how policies are introduced and enacted. Issue networks have replaced subgovernments as the forum within which policy discussions take place, implying that a much more diverse set of groups/actors is involved in deliberations and that the traditionally powerful interest groups will not prevail as frequently as was once the case. Dramatic changes in public policies occur when new ideas catch on, resulting in previously unexpected initiatives becoming new programs. This implies a merging of analytical discussions with political need, regardless of the arguments of interest groups. Finally, the increased activity of individual legislators and their staffs means that there are more potential avenues through which new initiatives will be introduced as specific policy suggestions to be debated and enacted.

The General Political Climate of the 1990s

Much of the political climate that affects health care policy is defined by what influences national policies. The national government provides most of the public dollars spent on health care delivery and determines many of the policies that influence state expenditures (especially through the Medicaid program). Therefore, this review of the current environment begins with the national government, and Congress in particular. State governments, however, are also important in the development of health care policy, so this section will include a discussion of the current policy environment in the states.

The decade of the 1990s began with contradictory messages concerning the possibility for new initiatives in public policy. The politics of enacting budgets that reduce the federal deficit dominated discussions in Congress, seemingly at the expense of any policy activities, including health initiatives. At the same time the problems in health care delivery and finance grow more serious, including the problem of how to provide access to care for the thirty-three million to thirty-eight million Americans who lack any form of health insurance. Although Congress has been reducing budgets in the Medicare program, it has also been expanding the Medicaid program by adding groups of persons to those eligible for benefits (such as all children in families with incomes below 135 percent of the federal poverty level). In 1990 the Pepper Commission published its report, which advocates a major new federal program to expand the availability of health care to those without insurance. Since the commission was divided on its recommendations (most of the principal recommendations were narrowly approved), the report itself may not be the blueprint for policies. It will serve, however, as a catalyst for a sharpened debate among a number of different proposals (even those members of Congress voting against the commission recommendations have approaches of their own to suggest).

Can new policy ideas surface and become programs in an era of budgetary constraints? There are two parts to an answer to this question. First, new ideas that are "budget neutral" (even if only in the first year) can be more easily adopted in this environment. Second, Congress was still active in 1991 in passing major authorization legislation despite the time and energy devoted to budget enactment.

The vehicle Congress has used since 1981 to achieve savings in the budget to stay within deficit targets[5] is reconciliation legislation, passed as an omnibus bill every year since 1981 except 1988 (the year President Reagan vowed not to sign either an Omnibus Reconciliation Act or a continuing resolution to keep the government functioning without enacting the thirteen appropriations bills). Reconciliation is a process whereby specific appropriation decisions are made

5. Congress defines the deficit targets according to the provisions of the Gramm-Rudman-Hollings deficit legislation but achieves "budget savings" by reducing *anticipated* spending, not current year expenditures (Wildavsky 1988).

that in total keep federal spending within targets determined by Congress. For example, if Congress sets a target for the Medicare program which necessitates reductions in future spending, reconciliation decisions would be made to determine how spending would be reduced. Those decisions appear in omnibus budget reconciliation acts, which can contain a large number of measures that are only loosely related to one another. Since the reconciliation legislation is "omnibus," provisions not necessarily designed to reduce deficit spending can be inserted.[6] This process provides an opportunity to introduce new ideas that change existing programs. Provisions related to Medicare in recent years have changed the reimbursement scheme to reduce the disparity between payments to urban and rural hospitals (1989); policies have been enacted to change delivery of care in nursing homes to meet new and more stringent quality standards (1986); and a new program to provide federal grants to rural hospitals to "transition" into a different configuration was enacted in reconciliation (1988). Reconciliation also offers an opportunity not overlooked by members of Congress to micromanage the administration of programs. For example, the Consolidated Omnibus Reconciliation Act of 1985 includes a section (9121) detailing the responsibilities of Medicare hospitals in emergency cases.

While not normally a vehicle for major new programs, reconciliation can be used to change dramatically the direction of public policies. Two important changes in health policy in recent years have both been enacted through reconciliation—a change to relative value-based reimbursement for physicians[7] and a major new federal initiative supporting efforts to establish acceptable protocols for specific medical procedures.

A more common vehicle for new programs remains the traditional route of authorization legislation. Major new health programs began by this route in the 1980s, one involving organ transplantation and another public health (preventive measures) programs. In 1988 Congress enacted the most sweeping change in the Medicare program's history—the Medicare Catastrophic Coverage Act; however, it was repealed one year later.

6. The provisions, then, do not have to be directly germane to the purpose of the legislation. Although this may be a violation of rules and/or intent, the practice was only questioned seriously in 1989, when Senator Mitchell, majority leader of the Senate, refused to allow amendments, but after realizing his own proposal would be subject to the same decision, he relented and another omnibus bill was passed with multiple provisions not directly related to deficit reduction.

7. Relative value–based reimbursement is a new method to pay physicians by an objective calculation of the value of their services; it is based on the time required, the cost to the physician, and the value of the training needed to perform the service.

The atmosphere of spending constraints in Congress may seem at first blush to be a severe limit on new initiatives in health policy. It actually creates new opportunities, however, through reconciliation legislation. The principal limitation is that of funding support for federal commitments. But within spending limits, new programs are possible—for example the one suggested by Democratic senators in 1991 to provide health insurance to more Americans by mandating coverage through private employers.

THE POLITICAL ENVIRONMENT IN THE STATES

Ronald Reagan began his presidency with an agenda that included turning over many responsibilities to the states that the national government had assumed, beginning with the Great Society programs of President Lyndon Johnson. President Reagan was not successful in decentralizing all the programs he listed, nor was his scheme of swapping federal responsibility for welfare programs with state responsibility for Medicaid successful. His philosophy of federalism, however, combined with the budget constraints facing the national government, created a political environment within which states are expected to address new problems or significant changes in policy approaches to existing problems.

These are not entirely new expectations for states; they have traditionally been the frontline players in domestic policy. What is different about the 1980s is the demand for state financing of the programs. Previously, especially as evidenced in the Great Society programs and federal revenue sharing, the federal government provided much of the financial support for program initiatives, whether they originated in state government or the federal bureaucracy. The burden of paying for programs makes it all the more difficult for states to act when dealing with difficult problems and creates the temptation to retrench rather than expand efforts in domestic policies, including health policy. The same biases at work in the federal government—protecting the budget from overcommitment—exist in the state governments.

Nevertheless, states have a difficult time turning a cold shoulder to the problems of their citizens. They are in a better position to take actions that are not necessarily costly, using their powers to regulate providers. Specifying a single political climate applicable to fifty states is impossible, but there has been a general trend to increased activity in health care issues in recent years as the federal role has diminished and new problems (or restatements of old ones) have emerged, such as resolving access problems in areas with no or insufficient numbers of health professionals. Opportunities are arising for policy entrepreneurship in state governments that parallel those in the federal government.

A few policy concerns illustrate the argument just presented. State governments have begun to enact policies to finance health care for the uninsured. Those policies range from mandated health insurance to extended Medicaid benefits to direct payments to hospitals providing uncompensated care. New policies to promote access to care among rural populations are emerging in state legislatures, ranging from creating offices of rural health to providing direct assistance to community hospitals. State governments are also in the forefront of providing new programs for special populations, such as new groups included in Medicaid programs and persons with AIDS. State programs combating the AIDS epidemic have benefited from the traditional mechanism of federal grants, especially since the Ryan White Comprehensive AIDS Resources Emergency Act of 1990 was implemented in October 1991. State governments are also active in the important arena of preventive health programs, through state departments of public health.

State governments are typically a source of innovative approaches in domestic polices, and the decade of the 1980s was a time of developing innovative approaches that are cost effective means of confronting the major issues facing states, including health care. The interesting question will be how states with different political traditions approach the health care delivery problems of the next decade.

Conclusion

A doomsayer could look at the fiscal problems facing many of the nation's states and the national government and conclude that the future is bleak, holding out little prospect for innovative policies designed to address problems of access to health care, improving quality of care being delivered, or adopting a new system for reimbursement that would require investment in administrative time and skills to implement. The discussion in this chapter, however, provides reasons to expect continued policy activity. The traditional political barriers to changes in health policy have eroded thanks to the evolution of a new issue network both nationally and in the separate states and to the emergence of new leaders who can take full advantage of the analysis produced by players in the issue network.

Because of the changes in the issue network and the increased premium placed on the products of policy analysis (for example, in the development of the prospective payment system and the forthcoming resource-based system for paying physicians), there is a greater possibility than previously to merge the concerns of access, quality, and cost containment into a coherent policy. That merger, however, is not likely to occur until more incremental policies have failed, particularly those that promise to improve access by covering additional groups of persons such as the employed-uninsured. Those policies will not yield universal access to health care any more than a new payment system for physicians will arrest the increases in total health expenditures. Those policies, and others that may be forthcoming, will pave the way for continued movement toward more drastic reform of the health care delivery system in the United States. Such reform, cast in the rhetoric and reality of national health insurance, may ultimately be the only means of assuring universal access to care without sacrificing quality and at the same time containing health care expenditures. Many health policy analysts would agree with Morone (1990b) that U.S. policymakers are sliding toward a national health plan to resolve what appears to be intractable problems. The next few chapters will focus on those major problems, and the last two chapters will examine the prospects for more sweeping change.

3

. . .

Government, Business, and
Issues of Payment

Health care expenditure increases have prompted concern among those who pay the bills that health care is becoming unaffordable. Both the costs of specific services and the total volume of services provided have increased dramatically since the early 1980s. Since government accounts for approximately 40 percent of national health expenditures, policymakers have been attempting to establish policies that at least contain health expenditure increases. Large private corporations and insurance companies are equally anxious to lower the burden of health care costs on their businesses and products. Publicity about the high comparative cost of U.S. and foreign products has increased awareness among the public that health care expenditures may be causing economic problems.

When the objective of public policies is to control *aggregate expenditures* rather than costs of particular services or fees charged by any particular group of providers, policies will need to affect the entire health care delivery system. In order to understand this principle, this chapter includes a section describing in some detail the nature of this system. Recent changes in the system will be highlighted.

The complexity of the delivery system is only half the reason effectively controlling expenditure increases will prove difficult. The other half is the complexity of the system of financing health care in the United States. Government payment policies will affect only a portion (albeit a large portion) of expenditures; the private sector continues to finance most health care expenditures in the United States. Unlike the government, where one payer (the federal government through Medicare and the states following that lead with Medicaid policies) determines reimbursement policies, the private sector includes a diverse group of insurers and corporations responsible for payment policy decisions.

The immediate objective of government cost containment policies is to control the expenditures incurred by government, not all health care expenditures. This seemingly modest objective is still difficult to achieve because expenditures can be shifted to a part of the health care delivery system not directly affected by the given policy. With changes in health care delivery, however, it may be possible to achieve cost savings that heretofore have not existed. New participants in issue networks concerned with health policy issues, including health care providers, may be more willing to accommodate changes in payment systems.

The Health Care Delivery System

The health care delivery system is a complex mosaic of individuals and organizations involved in selling goods and delivering services to individual consumers. The stereotypical notion of an individual physician providing all the care each person needs, either directly or in combination with specialists recommended by the primary care physician, represents the way many still view the system. The reality is that the primary care physician does not control all that happens in patient care. Institutional management is more important than ever in determining treatment modalities, and organizations increasingly influence even the decisions made by individual physicians.

INSTITUTIONS

Since the early twentieth-century, hospitals have been the preeminent health care institutions in the United States. Between 1873 and 1909, the number of hospitals in the country increased from 178 to 4,356, with 421,065 beds. The mission of hospitals expanded to include treating all patients, not just the indigent (Rosenberg 1979). Many voluntary hospitals at the turn of the century were receiving government assistance to complete their missions (Stevens 1982). As hospitals became a central focal point for the practice of medicine, control over hospital policy shifted from trustees to physicians with admitting privileges (Starr 1982a). Hospitals became the institutions wherein physicians practiced the most advanced treatments and where patients were admitted as a place in which to recover from illness (not a place of last resort when illnesses progressed beyond the ability of medicine to handle them).

Two other indicators provide evidence of the growing importance of hospitals. First, the percentage of health care expenditures devoted to services provided in hospitals increased from 18 percent in 1929 to 40 percent in 1980 (Temin 1988). Second, the number of inpatient and outpatient visits grew from 20 million in 1950 to 360 million in 1990 (Donham et al. 1991). Hospitals became the preferred practice site for expensive procedures.

Two important shifts have occurred in the hospital industry in recent years: an increasing number of hospitals are associated with nationwide chains, and hospital services are shifting from reliance on inpatient care to increased use of outpatient services and other programs. Between 1975 and 1982, the percentage of American hospitals affiliated with multihospital systems increased from 25 percent to 33 percent. Most of the growth occurred between 1975 and 1979; affiliation activity slowed between 1980 and 1982 (Ermann and Gabel 1984). The growth in systems and alliances has increased again in recent years; by 1985 systems "owned, leased or sponsored 1,885 hospitals and managed, under contract, 595 hospitals" (Wacker, Reczynski, and Tibbs 1987). By 1990, the number of for-profit hospitals had increased to 749, representing over 11 percent of all hospitals in the United States (American Hospital Association 1991). In 1988, the top twenty-five investor-owned hospital management companies owned and/or managed 1,394 hospitals in the United States. (Leberto 1988). In addition to investor-owned companies, nonprofit alliances have grown rapidly in popularity. The two largest alliances, Voluntary Hospitals of America and American Healthcare Systems, grew from 483 hospitals combined in 1984 to 1,059 in 1986 (Wacker, Reczynski, and Tibbs 1987).

The growth in multihospital chains has two important implications. First, management efficiencies may be realized as a result of negotiated agreements and sharing managerial talent. This is an especially important benefit to those hospitals joining the two large alliances. Second, to the extent the proprietary chains gain new members, more hospitals will be explicitly seeking profits to be shared with owners of the chains. As recently as 1984, investor-owned chains owned or managed fewer than 1,000 hospitals (Wacker, Reczynski, and Tibbs 1987), compared to the nearly 1,400 hospitals now included in the top twenty-five investor-owned systems. Some commentators have long criticized the emphasis on profit inherent in proprietary ownership, saying it is inappropriate in the delivery of medical care (Relman 1980). As a result of the concern about the relationship of the profit motive to the delivery of health care, the Institute of Medicine (IOM) in 1986 published a major study, *For-profit Enterprise in Health Care* (Washington, D.C.: National Academy Press). It found that proprietary institutions provided far less charity care than did nonprofits but that the overall quality of the care delivered was the same. The IOM recommended continued monitoring of the care delivered by these organizations. The IOM also called for continued physician influence in hospital management decisions, lest patient welfare be sacrificed to corporate profits (Gray and McNerney 1986).

Researchers have found some basic differences between proprietary and nonprofit hospitals. Watt and colleagues concluded, based on studies of hospitals in 1978 and 1980, that investor-owned hospitals were more profitable, a result principally of more aggressive pricing strategies and not greater management efficiencies (Watt et al. 1986). After reviewing a number of studies, Sloan (1988) concluded that differences in efficiencies are small across hospitals of different ownership, that there is little difference in the profitability of specific services offered, that for-profit hospitals are less likely to engage in medical education, and that for-profit hospitals are less likely to finance charity care. His general conclusion is that there is little difference among hospitals of different ownership type.

The question of what differences there might be between for-profit and nonprofit hospitals remains an important one. As changes occur in the basis of hospital payment, hospitals with different economic motives may react differently. The for-profit hospitals can be expected to continue to maintain profit maximization as their principal objective and adjust management practices accordingly. Nonprofits may react by increasing their reliance on external sources of revenue, such as trust funds and local taxes, while allowing fiscal deficits to increase. This reaction will receive greater consideration when the topic of payment policy is discussed more fully.

All hospitals have been changing the mixture of services they offer, increasing outpatient care that does not require overnight admission to the hospital. The following numbers compare the percentage of hospitals providing these services in 1985 and 1990: outpatient departments, 50 and 84 percent, alcoholism and chemical dependency outpatient programs, 15 and 20 percent; outpatient rehabilitation programs, 38 and 50 percent; and outpatient psychiatric programs, 15 and 20 percent (American Hospital Association 1991). Programs have been increased that take hospital personnel into the community, such as home health care services, which 30 percent of the nation's hospitals offered in 1985, compared to 15 percent in 1983 (Wacker et. al. 1987); by 1990 that percentage grew to nearly 36 percent (American Hospital Association 1991). During the 1980s, hospitals were increasingly performing surgeries on an outpatient rather than inpatient basis; increasing from 24 percent of hospitals doing so in 1983 to 40 percent in 1986 (American Hospital Association 1987).

Changes in hospital services have occurred in response to changes in payment systems, treatment modalities, and competition from other providers. Insurance carriers and large employers have, in recent years, attempted to limit the amount of money spent for hospital care by reducing utilization of inpatient hospital facilities. Hospitals have adjusted by offering other services. The shift away from inpatient services has been facilitated by changes in how certain illnesses are treated by medical professionals. Certain surgical procedures that once required hospitalization can now be performed without admitting the patient to the hospital for an overnight stay. For example, breast biopsies no longer require inpatient admission. Such changes have allowed institutions other than hospitals to offer surgical procedures, and the response of hospitals has been to increase the number and use of outpatient surgery units.

Proprietary ownership is common in the second major health care institution to be described here—nursing homes. Of the approximately 19,100 nursing homes nationally, nearly 15,000 are owned and operated by private, for-profit firms (Bishop 1988). Just over 40 percent of all homes are members of multiple institution groups (Bishop 1988). For public policy, the most crucial homes are those that serve Medicare and Medicaid patients. Of the 7,379 skilled nursing facilities certified for Medicare and Medicaid, 66 percent are proprietary institutions, 22 percent are nonprofit institutions, and 12 percent are government owned (Bureau of Data Management and Strategy, 1988).

Nursing homes are important institutions in the development of long-term care policy, which will be addressed in chapter 5. They are not the only institutions providing such care, however. There has been a recent and rapid growth in the number of home health care agencies that provide long-term care. The number of agencies grew 25 percent from 1984 to 1985 alone, numbering 5,343 in 1985 (Riffer 1985). By 1988, the number of home health agencies certified by Medicare grew to 5,769 (Bureau of Data Management and Strategy 1988). Whether provided in a nursing home or in private homes by home health agencies, long-term care promises to be a growth service into the next century, given the aging of the baby-boom population. By 1990, nursing home care already accounted for $53.1 billion in health care expenditures, and home health care another $6.9 billion (Levit et al. 1991). Costs of caring for the elderly with moderate to severe dementia are estimated to be $35.8 billion per year and may increase to $80 billion annually by 2010 (Cassel et al. 1992).

Hospitals and nursing homes are the major institutional actors providing medical care services. Other institutions providing services include laboratories, pharmacies, hospices, and various clinics. The total share of health care expenditures devoted to those institutions is quite small, but they can be important in particular policy concerns. For example, more than 500 rural health clinics are important in considering how to expand access to health care in remote regions of the country. As another example, the presence of ambulatory surgical centers creates competitive pressure to help control prices for outpatient surgical procedures. There are two important conclusions to be reached about health care institutions. First, they are in some instances substitutable (freestanding surgical facilities and hospitals), which means that policies can take advantage of competitive forces. Second, they are in other instances complementary (rural health clinics that extend care to remote regions), which means that policies can extend the reach of health care services to otherwise excluded populations.

INDIVIDUAL PROVIDERS

There are several groups of providers involved in delivering health care; policy issues include assuring a sufficient number and desirable geographic distribution of each. Each group of providers has, over the years, become increasingly professional and specialized. For example, many nurses now have baccalaureate preparation rather than shorter nursing training programs, and many now receive advanced degrees. As groups of providers become more knowledgeable about diagnosis and treatment, some become substitutable for others. For example, physician's assistants are qualified to complete medical histories, make some diagnoses, and provide limited treatment. The growth of medical professions and numbers of persons who practice them creates both problems and opportunities for policymakers. The following discussion of each group in turn will develop that theme.

The preeminent individual provider in health care is the physician, and there were 615,421 of them in 1990, or 244 per 100,000 population. There was an 18 percent increase in the number of physicians between 1980 and 1986, and a 13 percent increase in the number per 100,000 population for those same years. In 1986 there were 462,126 physicians involved in patient care (Robach et al. 1992). Table 3.1 shows the seven largest classifications of physicians, categorized by the number of practicing professionals for each specialty.

A debate continues over whether or not the nation will experience a physician surplus in the next twenty years. As stated above, the number of physicians

Table 3.1 Active Physicians by Specialty, 1986

Specialty	Number of Physicians
Internal Medicine	91,333
Family Practice	42,497
Pediatrics	36,518
Psychiatry	32,724
Obstretrics/Gynecology	31,364
General Practice	25,190

Source: *Physician Characteristics and Distribution in the United States*. Chicago: American Medical Association, 1987.

has been increasing, and the ratio of physicians to the general population has improved in the past ten years. There remains some concern, however, that the number of general and family practice physicians (the "family doctor") is insufficient. Whereas in 1970 over 21 percent of physicians were general practitioners, by 1986 that had shrunk to 14.3 percent (Bureau of Data Management and Strategy 1988). When the ratio of physicians per 100,000 population in the United States is compared to the same ratio for Canada, the United States does not fare well in providing primary care physicians. The U.S. ratio for general/family practice is only 28 per 100,000, compared to 89 in Canada. By contrast, the U.S. ratio for all specialties is consistently higher than that in Canada.

A complete discussion of the appropriate number of physicians includes careful consideration of the demand for medical care. It will increase as the population ages and uncomplicated conditions are treated in a timely and effective manner, leaving more persons susceptible to complicated conditions. The work habits of physicians, including the number of hours per week worked and the number of patients seen per hour of work, affect the ability of supply to satisfy demand. Finally, the role of other personnel in taking over tasks formerly performed by physicians could expand supply relative to demand. After statistical consideration of these factors, some researchers are concluding that there will be a continued need for more physicians into the next century (Schwartz, Sloan, and Mendelson 1988; Schloss 1988; and Hanft 1987). One study, after adjusting for physicians not entering the practice of medicine, differences between practice styles of male and female physicians (who are an increasing percentage of new physicians), and changes in productivity, projected more than 100,000 fewer physicians by the year 2000 than did the 1980 report of the Graduate Medical Education National Advisory Committee (Jacobsen and Rimm 1987).

The debate over the supply of physicians is an important public policy issue because policy decisions influence the number of persons entering the medical profession and because that number in turn has implications for other policies. The number of new entrants into the profession is influenced by programs of government assistance for individual students and by government assistance given directly to institutions. An increased supply of physicians may result in increased health care expenditures because of increased demand for care induced by the physicians and/or the substitution of physician treatment for less expensive modalities. An increased supply of physicians may also help alleviate shortages in certain regions of the country.

Physicians are no longer characteristically self-employed in a solo practice. From 1983 to 1988 the percentage of physicians practicing in solo offices fell from 40.5 percent to 38.5 percent, even though 76.6 percent of physicians were still self-employed (Marder et al. 1988). A large number of self-employed physicians are affiliated with groups of doctors, commonly through an individual practice association (a form of health maintenance organization) or as part of a preferred provider organization (PPO, an arrangement providing price breaks to large purchasers).

The continued increases in group practice environments, with nonphysician administrators controlling management decisions, troubles many physicians. Like any other professionals, physicians want control over their own working environments, including working conditions and determining their own incomes (Feldstein, 1977). Physicians working in health maintenance organizations (HMOs) are especially likely to sacrifice at least some degree of professional autonomy to pressures to adopt cost-efficient practice styles. This creates conflict between professionals and organizations and an incentive for physicians to become more knowledgeable about the economic consequences of their decisions (Kralewski et al. 1987). They may develop organizations of their own to achieve greater collective power.

There is even a possibility that physicians' unions will gain popularity. As of 1985, there were unions in eight states, with a total membership of 25,000 (Colburn 1985). The formation of unions is most likely in hospitals and HMOs, where there may be large groups of physicians subject to the same management decisions. The combination of increased use of group practices and increases in government and third-party conditions on payment has been cited by some as proof of a dramatic loss of control by physicians. McKinlay and Arches (1985) have argued that physicians are in effect becoming governed by bureaucracies

48

and that therefore we are witnessing the "proletarianization of physicians." Stevens (1986) extends that argument by arguing that the physicians of the future will be employed in a corporate environment, affecting how they approach their jobs: "Significantly, he/she will be assessed not only on technical and behavioral skills but on conformance to the prevailing corporate 'style,' corporate goals, and corporate ethos" (Stevens 1986, 79).

What are the implications of these changes in the role of the physician in the economics of health care delivery? Thus far, physician income has not been affected. Real income among all physicians increased from $75,000 in 1981 to $92,000 in 1988 (Gonzales 1989). Table 3.2 shows the nominal incomes for selected specialties. Although real income has increased for physicians in recent years, the ability of each physician to act as an autonomous player in the health care arena is eroding. Because increasing numbers of physicians are members of groups, there may be a greater potential for policy initiatives to influence actions taken by physicians. Negotiated agreements can be struck with groups of physicians.

In recent years the roles of other health care providers have achieved new significance as policymakers sought solutions to problems of expanding access to care and containing health care expenditures. Physician extenders are often viewed as alternative providers of choice in remote areas and in all areas for a limited array of services performed more inexpensively by persons who charge less than physicians. They include nurse midwives, nurse practitioners, physician's assistants, and nurse anesthetists. As of 1985 there were 16,757 registered nurse midwives and nurse practitioners, 19,070 clinical nurses, and 13,000 physician's assistants (Heinrich 1985). Although these personnel normally work under the direct supervision of physicians, recent initiatives in state laws have begun to permit practice under indirect supervision. Physician's assistants and nurse practitioners, for example, can staff clinics in communities unable to recruit physicians. Continuing to expand the roles of alternative providers promises to be a major policy concern for state governments in the next few years. Physicians can be expected to object to extensive changes in laws governing scope of practice, since those changes could result in substitute labor for what were previously their tasks (Feldstein 1977).

Another major category of health provider is general nursing. Policymakers have turned attention to nursing in recent years because of a shortage of nurses, particularly in hospitals. During 1989 more than 75 percent of the hospitals in the Unites States reported nursing shortages; 30 percent of urban hospitals

Table 3.2 Income of Physicians by Specialty, 1988 (In Thousands of Dollars, Pretaxes)

Specialty	Income
General/Family Practice	85
Internal Medicine	109
Surgery	180
Pediatrics	85
Obstretrics/Gynecology	150
Radiology	158
Psychiatry	97
Anesthesiology	180
Pathology	130

Source: Gonzales 1989

and 15 percent of rural hospitals closed beds during 1987 because of the shortage (Aiken 1989). According to a report by the U.S. Department of Health and Human Services, we can anticipate a shortage of 343,000 nurses by the year 2000 (Fowler 1987). Nurses are used by hospitals because of their flexibility to perform a variety of tasks in those institutions; as hospitalized patients require more intensive care the need for nurses has increased. Filling hospital vacancies and relying on nurses for duties will require increased incentives to induce persons to enter and remain in this profession. Those incentives might include better working conditions (hours per week and more control over tasks performed), increased salaries, and increased benefits (Demkovich 1987).

The theme of this discussion of institutions and providers is that substitution is increasingly possible, of one type of institution for another and of one type of professional for another.[1] A final possibility for substitution must be considered—the use of different mechanisms for contracting for services. The most popular of those is to use HMOs; rapidly growing in popularity is the use of preferred provider organizations (PPOs).

The use of HMOs dates from the early creation of the Kaiser plans in California following World War II. As a reform of the delivery system they became well known following their promotion by the Richard Nixon presidential administration and the enactment of the Health Maintenance Organization Act of

1. This discussion of health care professionals has focused on those providing acute medical care. Dentists, hygienists, and others involved in more specialized care of patients have been omitted for the purposes of parsimony. They are part of the health care delivery system but not a part of the system that is often the object of attention of policymakers at all levels of government; the providers discussed in this chapter fit those criteria.

1973. In 1970 there were thirty-seven HMOs, with sixteen in California, and 67 percent of all HMOs were in western states (Gruber, Shader, and Polich 1988). At Nixon's urging, the federal government encouraged further development of HMOs by providing planning and start-up funding for new HMOs. By 1980, the federal government had contributed $190 million through this program (Gruber, Shader, and Polich 1988). The program, however, was plagued by problems caused by compromises struck in order to secure congressional action. Specifically, HMOs were required to provide a complete array of services for a single community rate. As a result early federally assisted HMOs had difficulty developing cost-effective plans. Other carriers, particularly private firms other than Blue Cross, were basing insurance premiums on the experiences of particular groups, often employers with histories of relatively less health care use. These premiums, based on experience rating, were less than those charged by HMOs using community rating.

In 1976, the HMO Act was amended in an attempt to liberalize the qualifications necessary for funding, resulting in a doubling in the number of federally assisted HMOs from 42 in 1977 to 79 in 1978 (Gruber, Shader, and Polich 1988). By the mid 1980s, at the urging of President Reagan, federal financial support for HMOs dwindled. By then, however, the number of federally qualified HMOs exceeded 300, and in 1987 there were 662 HMOs (data from 1986 and 1987 presented in Gruber, Shader, and Polich 1988). The number of HMOs fell to 590 in 1989, but the number of enrollees increased to nearly 32.5 million after a 1.7 percent increase in the first half of the year (Interstudy 1989). In four states (California, Oregon, Minnesota, and Massachusetts), at least 25 percent of the population is enrolled in HMOs (*HealthWeek,* 17 June 1991).

HMOs come in three different varieties. Staff model HMOs employ physicians as salaried employees of an organization that both insures consumers for all their health care needs and provides for most of those needs in a single clinical environment. Group model HMOs also insure patients for all their care and employ physicians full-time as HMO providers but as a contract with their group rather than as salaried employees. Individual practice association (IPA) HMOs contract with private practicing providers to treat HMO patients (the contracts are usually on a per-patient per-month basis). The physicians treat other patients in their practices—their involvement with the HMO is on a specific patient-by-patient basis. Nearly two-thirds of all HMOs are the IPA model, whereas 51 percent of enrollees are in group model HMOs (Gruber, Shader, and Polich 1988).

HMOs have been attractive to groups because of potential cost savings resulting from a different style of practicing medicine. The management philosophy of an HMO is to retain as much patient care as possible within the outpatient environment, where the HMO's providers have maximum control over the volume and price of services rendered. Primary care physicians paid by the HMO become gatekeepers, determining any needs for specialist treatment. Without their specific referral, patients are not reimbursed for care outside of the HMO. The primary care physician is both the advocate for the patient and the protector of the organization's economic interests (Reagan 1987).

The net result of the different practice style is a reduction in medical procedures, especially those requiring hospitalization. Researchers using a carefully controlled design comparing HMO users to others concluded that the HMOs provide less expensive care (Manning et al. 1984). Over time, however, the cost advantage of the HMO could evaporate if the managed care approach spreads to other providers as well. Further, HMOs may experience greater costs as their member populations age (initial members are generally enrolled through an employer-based group health plan and are therefore relatively young at the time of enrollment). In short, there are forces driving health care expenditures that are beyond the control of HMOs.

A recent survey of employers reflects an awareness that HMOs will not necessarily control costs indefinitely. When presented with the statement that HMOs are effective in controlling costs, only 33 percent of employers agreed, and 32 percent disagreed. Fifty-two percent agreed with the statement that HMOs attract the better risks from the employee population (*Managed Health Care* 1989). Employers are becoming increasingly skeptical about HMOs, given recent premium increases for those plans; however, "HMOs cost employers significantly less than indemnity insurance, and workers are offered a broader package of benefits" (Firshein 1990).

HMOs are only one of a number of managed care options offered through private insurers. In 1986, HMOs accounted for 18 percent of group health plans, unmanaged fee-for-service accounted for 28 percent, managed fee-for-service 43 percent, and preferred provider organizations (PPOs) 11 percent (deLissovoy et al. 1987). Managed fee-for-service plans are those that require some review of cases before hospital costs will be reimbursed. Unmanaged fee-for-service plans are the traditional indemnity plans, which reimburse partially for all care and the choice of providers is left to the consumer. PPOs are arrangements between the insurer and a select group of providers who agree to provide health care services for a fee less than the normal market rate. PPOs have been an attractive option for both providers and insurers. Providers secure a steady flow of patients into what are still individual practices, while insurers gain some control over costs through negotiations with the providers. In 1984 there were 1.3 million persons enrolled in PPOs, by 1986 that number grew to 16.5 million, and in 1989 an estimated 18.3 million persons were enrolled in 678 PPOs (Marion Laboratories 1989).

SUMMARY

The growth of managed care plans is another indicator of the volatility in the health care delivery system. A number of alternative delivery mechanisms have been developed, and practice styles used in the direct delivery of care have changed considerably in recent years. The development of for-profit firms has complicated both the economics and politics of health care delivery. Physicians are no longer the private entrepreneurs of yesteryear; they often find themselves the employees of larger firms or participants in networks of physicians providing care to groups of persons on a contract basis. There are an increasing number of alternatives to physician care, including using allied health professionals for tasks not requiring the advanced training of medical doctors.

The changes in the delivery system create new opportunities for purchasers of health care services to gain some control over expenditures. The enrollments in HMOs and PPOs are at least in part attributable to this reality. Insurers, employers, and government may even be so bold as to refuse to pay for some treatments, knowing that less expensive alternatives are available. For example, many employers require precertification before hospitalization so that expensive hospital stays can be avoided when the same results can be accomplished on an outpatient basis. In short, policies governing payment for health care are changing rapidly, as is the delivery system.

Health Care Costs

All of us who have seen bills for health care, regardless of who will pay the bill, are aware of the high costs for this care. But are those costs too high? Are health care expenses somehow more outrageously high when compared to other expenses? If so, why?

Judging the relative value of any good is an iffy proposition, especially when the good or service is labor intensive. How much is a physician's labor worth? Several factual issues must be considered. We need to examine just how much health care costs, both as a total amount and for major components of that total (doctors, hospitals, use of advanced equipment, nursing homes, prescription medicine). We should also keep in mind specifically who pays the bill for health care, both as the first payer and the ultimate payer. Then we can render more reasoned judgment as to the burden imposed.

Once such judgment has been reached, and assuming we conclude the burden is too much, what do we do about it? The answer to this question also requires careful deliberation. We must first examine the evidence about why the costs are as high as they are. After reaching some conclusions concerning causes we can develop solutions. A preliminary word of caution is in order. We will not be able to avoid trade-offs in agreeing to such conclusions. Because we cannot state with complete certainty the reasons for the costs, we will not be certain that in reducing expenses we do not also reduce the quality of, and access to, care. As described above, the medical care delivery system includes a complex set of interactions among many actors; pressure in one part of that system has implications for the entire system. Therefore, a cost-containment policy may be effective in reducing expenditures for inpatient hospital treatment, but ineffective in reducing total expenditures because treatment sites shift to other locations.

In 1990, $666 billion was spent on health care in the United States, or 12.2 percent of the gross national product (Levit et al. 1991). During 1989, medical care prices rose 8.5 percent, versus a 4.6 percent increase for general prices in the economy (*Medicine & Health* 1990). That disparity in growth rates continued throughout 1991 and into 1992, as displayed in figure 3.1, which shows the monthly increases in health expenditures and the consumer price index. Total health expenditures for 1991 have been estimated to be $738 billion, or about 13 percent of the GNP (U.S. Commerce Department estimates). When expenditures reach these levels, money is not available for other uses.

For individuals, health care expenditures are high but not always noticed. In 1990 an average of $2,566 was spent on personal health care for each person in the nation. Direct patient payments, however, accounted for only 21 percent of all sources of payment for health care. Private health insurance carriers paid 33 percent of the health care bill that year, whereas government (through Medicare, Medicaid, and other programs) contributed 41 percent. The remaining 4 percent was paid from other private sources (such as private foundations that support local hospitals) (Levitt et al. 1991). In another, more startling view of individual and household expenditures for health care, the average household spent $8,000 in 1990 for a variety of health care expenditures, including payroll taxes, general taxes that support health programs, and reduced wages to support benefits (Urban Institute report referenced in *Medicine & Health* 1992).

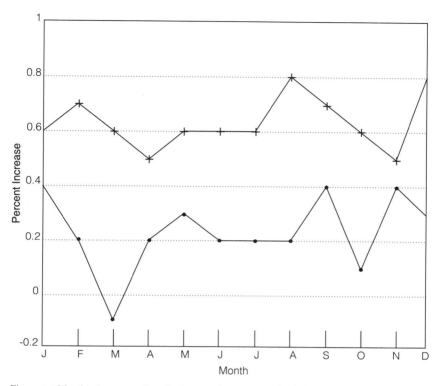

Figure 3.1 Monthly increases of medical care and consumer price index, 1991. From *Medicine & Health,* vol. 45, Jan.–Dec. 1991.

Are health care expenditures rising too rapidly? They are certainly outpacing general price increases, as specified above. Another clear indication of the disproportionate increases in health care expenditures, compared to overall price increases, is to track health expenditures as a percentage of gross national product. Figure 3.2 shows the percent of GNP spent for health care in each year from 1980 through 1990.

Are health expenditure increases justified because the cost of providing care has increased this rapidly? We can test this notion by examining the factors that account for the increase (this is separate from the examination of the causes of the total cost, which will come later in this chapter). General inflation accounted for 65 percent of the increase in health expenditures between 1988 and 1989, but 21 percent was the result of prices unique to the health care system increasing rapidly from one year to the next. During the decade of the 1980s, medical-specific inflation in excess of inflation in the general economy caused

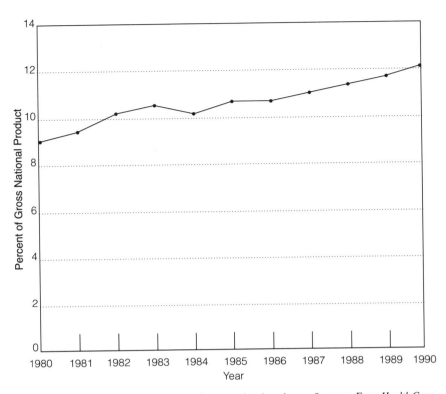

Figure 3.2 Health expenditures as percent of gross national product, 1980–1990. From *Health Care Financing Review* 8, no. 1, Fall 1986 and vol. 13, no. 1, Fall 1991.

22 percent of the growth in the cost for medical services (Levit et al. 1991, 30). This is the contributing factor most often highlighted in policy discussions—these price increases often seem to be arbitrary efforts by providers to increase their incomes more rapidly than justified. Of the balance of the increase from 1988 to 1989, 9 percent was the result of population growth and 26 percent the result of such factors as the increase in the elderly population, increased consumption per capita, and changes in the types of services (Lazenby and Letsch 1990).

Figure 3.3 summarizes the information concerning reasons for increases in health expenditures. To say these explanations exist, however, is not to say that costs could not be contained. Did consumption have to increase? Did changing the types of services have to result in higher prices? These questions will be answered in the context of a political system. If there is sufficient public pressure to do something about the high cost of health care, the answers will be no.

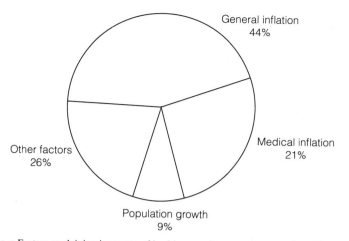

Figure 3.3 Factors explaining increases of health expenditures as percent of total increase. From Lazenby and Letsch 1990.

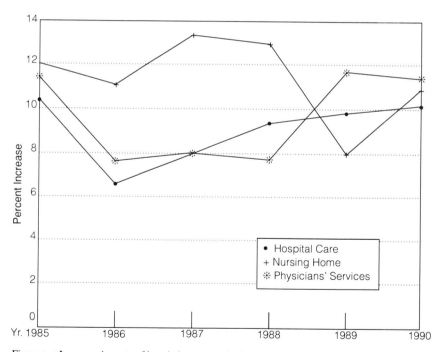

Figure 3.4 Increases in costs of hospital care, nursing home care, and physicians' services, 1985–1990. From Levit et al. 1991.

Table 3.3 Health Care Expenditures by Major Category, Selected Years (In Billions of Dollars)

	1970	1975	1980	1985	1986	1987	1988	1989	1990
All Health Expenditures	74.4	132.9	250.1	422.6	452.3	492.5	546.0	602.8	666.2
Hospital Care	27.9	52.4	102.4	168.3	179.4	193.8	212.0	232.6	256.0
Physicians' Services	13.6	23.3	41.9	74.0	82.1	93.0	105.1	113.6	125.7
Drugs and Nondurables	8.8	13.0	21.6	36.2	35.6	38.7	46.3	50.6	54.6
Nursing Home Care	4.9	9.9	20.0	34.1	36.7	29.8	42.8	47.7	53.1

Source: Health Care Financing Administration, Office of the Actuary, reported in *Health Care Financing Review,* Winter 1990 and Fall 1991.

A complete understanding of the costs of health care requires knowing how the health care dollar is divided among the various components of the system. As discussed earlier, the system is a menagerie of various providers, but the most costly ones are hospital care, physicians' services, dentists' services, other professional services, drugs, eyeglasses and appliances, and nursing home care. Table 3.3 shows expenditures for hospital care, nursing home care, physicians' services, and drugs and nondurables, 1970–89. Figure 3.4 shows graphically the annual increases in expenditures for hospital care, nursing home care, and physicians' services, 1985–90. Figure 3.5 shows the distribution of the health care dollar among the major categories in 1990.

Quite obviously, hospital care accounts for the greatest share of all expenses (39 percent), whereas physicians account for 19 percent. Lest we believe, however, that physicians are not the principal generators of health care costs, consider what they do in the course of their practices. Physicians hospitalize patients and release them from hospitals. Admission and length-of-stay decisions are controlled by doctors, which means that some portion of the 39 percent of health expenditures consumed by hospitals must be attributed to physician preference for treatments. Of course, physicians cannot control what a hospital room costs, and that charge has increased dramatically in recent years. Nor do they control the costs of procedures that rely on using expensive equipment. They do, however, control what the procedures will be for each case whether or not a patient is admitted a day before procedures are scheduled.

As the largest single source of health care expenditures, hospitals were the

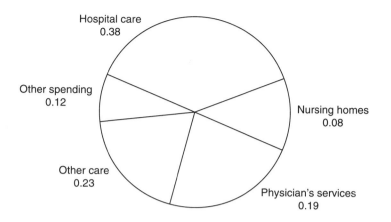

Figure 3.5 Allocation of the health dollar, 1990. From Levit et al. 1991.

focus of cost-containment policies in the 1980s. Policies were enacted to pressure hospital managers to keep costs below predetermined spending limits and help modify the behavior of other actors in the delivery system, physicians in particular. At least in part because of new incentives, the site for much medical care shifted from inpatient hospital to outpatient settings (Levit and Freeland 1988). Figure 3.6 shows the annual changes in the number of hospital admissions and the number of outpatient visits, 1977 through 1987.

Have these behavioral changes resulted in cost containment? Hospital expenditure increases slowed in the mid- and late 1980s (Letsch, Levit, and Waldo 1988). They increased at the end of the decade, however, 8.6 percent in 1988 and 9.1 percent in 1989, and again in 1990, 9.5 percent (Kimball 1990). The increases are explained by the increased use of expensive procedures in hospitals and by a shift to outpatient care in hospitals. Outpatient revenue for hospitals increased 11.7 percent over annual increases for inpatient revenue (Kimball 1990). Expenditures for professional services grew rapidly throughout the 1980s and continued to do so into the 1990s.

Federal government efforts to contain hospital expenditures have had a modest impact on federal spending through the Medicare program. From an annual increase of 21.4 percent in 1984, Medicare payments to hospitals grew only 5.2 percent in 1986 and 8 percent in 1988. These payments include outpatient services and hospital-based home health agencies, which are not subject to the strictures of the prospective payment system (Lazenby and Letsch 1990). Al-

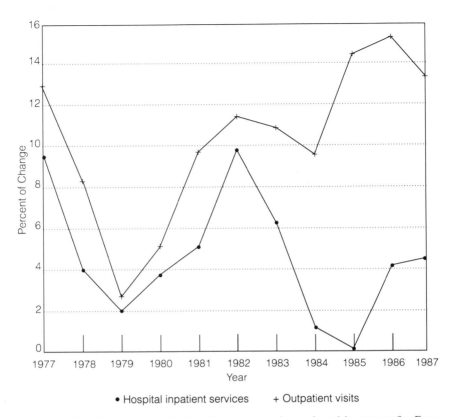

Figure 3.6 Annual change in hospital inpatient services and outpatient visits, 1977–1987. From Levit and Freeland 1988.

though there may have been a short term decline in hospital payments in the Medicare program, however, long-term trends still indicate rising expenditures. Figure 3.4 plots the annual expenditure changes in hospital care, physicians' services, and nursing home care for selected years since 1965. The resulting graph demonstrates the return of cost escalation since 1986.

Cost-containment policies include physicians, especially the 1989 congressional action to implement a new payment scheme in Medicare (discussed in greater detail in chapters 4 and 6). In 1990, direct expenditures for physician care accounted for 21 percent of total health care expenditures (Levit et al. 1991, 33). They were expected to increase by 15 percent in 1990, following two years of 13 percent growth (Kimball 1990). Several major factors contribute to the increase in physician fees, including use, intensity of services, and prices charged for services (Division of National Cost Estimates 1987).

Other expenditures for health care are not current targets for major cost containment efforts, although their time may be coming. In 1989 personal health care expenditures other than physician care (including dental care, drugs, and eyeglasses) accounted for 23 percent of health expenditures and nursing homes 9 percent (Lazenby and Letsch 1990). Of those expenditures, the most likely subjects for public policy discussion in the near future are nursing homes and drugs. The Medicare Catastrophic Care Act of 1988 included provisions for Medicare payment for prescription medicine. It also created a commission similar to the Physician Payment Review Commission and the Prospective Payment Review Commission to study payment rates and other issues related to prescription medications. Nursing home expenditures are currently under review in many state governments, since approximately one half of all Medicaid costs are nursing home expenditures.

An important explanation for continued increases in health care expenditures is that the burden of payment is spread throughout society, such that very few persons directly confront the high costs of health care. Individuals and families do pay for some care with their personal incomes, usually as deductibles (a set amount paid before insurance becomes effective) and as copayments (a percentage of the total charges). Even though those costs have risen in recent years, they still represent, for most persons, only a small portion of the total costs. Similarly, there are some health care services (for example, routine office visits) that some insurance policies exclude from coverage, but they too represent a small portion of health care charges. Without a direct financial confrontation between the purchaser and the provider, little pressure exists to reduce the burden of payment. Most direct payment for health care services comes from government and private insurance carriers. Figure 3.7 shows the contributions from various sources of payment for health care in 1990. Direct payment from patients accounts for 25 percent of total payments, compared to 32 percent from private health insurance, and 41 percent from government sources (including Medicare and Medicaid). Payment has shifted from individuals to third parties in the past thirty years. In 1950, patients paid 83 percent of the bill themselves, whereas insurance paid 11.4 percent and government contributed very little (Medicare and Medicaid were enacted in 1965; until then government spending was limited). In 1967, patient direct share was down to 50 percent and insurance had increased its share to 29 percent. Government, now in the early years of Medicare and Medicaid, had increased its share to 20 percent. Table 3.4 shows

61

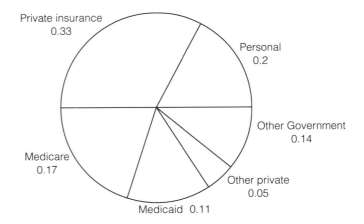

Private insurance 0.33

Personal 0.2

Other Government 0.14

Other private 0.05

Medicaid 0.11

Medicare 0.17

Figure 3.7 Funding of the health care dollar, 1990. From Levit et al. 1991.

the distribution of the payment sources for health care for the years 1970–1990. The trend away from direct patient payments has continued.

With aggregate health expenditures as high as they are in the United States, the argument that the absence of a classic supplier-purchaser relationship explains rapid expenditure increases is not entirely satisfying. Population growth contributes to increased health expenditures, particularly the growth during recent years in the number of elderly Americans and the oldest (over seventy-five years of age) of them, who are more likely to be heavy users of health care services. The costs of technology also contribute to high health care expenditures. Both diagnosis and treatment are improved by using the latest technological advances which are often expensive. Technology may be the major force driving health expenditures ever higher. New technological developments increase the number and costs of services available, and they make some procedures less invasive, which will increase use (Aaron 1991). More is involved here than exotic procedures such as organ transplants. Technological advances in diagnosis, such as magnetic resonance imaging, are quite costly but very helpful in confirming diagnoses. Antibiotics and other medicine can also be considered technological advances, and the costs involved in using them can be substantial. We may not require all of the technologies developed in recent years, particularly those which do not contribute significantly to sustaining a desirable quality of life.

The issue of oversupply is broader than just increasing numbers of techno-

Table 3.4 Distribution of Health Care Expenditures by Source of Payment, Selected Years, 1970–1990 (Percent of Total)

Source of Payment	1970	1975	1980	1985	1986	1987	1988	1989	1990
Out of Pocket	34.4	29.0	23.4	21.8	21.5	21.3	21.2	20.7	20.4
Private Insurance	22.4	24.8	29.5	31.9	31.7	31.7	32.4	33.1	32.5
Other Private	5.9	4.7	4.9	4.6	4.4	4.4	4.5	4.4	4.9
Federal Government	23.8	27.4	28.9	29.4	29.3	29.1	28.8	28.9	29.0
State & Local Government	13.3	14.1	13.3	12.3	13.0	13.4	13.1	13.0	13.0

Source: Health Care Financing Administration, Office of the Actuary, reported in *Health Care Financing Review,* Winter 1989, Winter 1990, and Fall 1991.

logical advances. We may have too many physicians (especially among some surgical specialties) in this country, and we certainly have too many hospital beds. Those who invested in careers and institutions will want to recover the costs of their investments. Therefore, the health care system has a tendency to create demand as needed to provide income for all in the system. Providers are in a position to do so. This is a strong indictment of the system, but there is evidence to support it. A great deal of research has been done on the variation in rates of surgery around the country, and the results are revealing. The likelihood for women at age 70 to have undergone a hysterectomy varies from 20 percent to 70 percent in Maine hospitals. In Vermont hospitals the probabilities for tonsillectomies varies from 40 to 70 percent (Wennberg 1986). These variations are due in large part to uncertainty about appropriate treatment and to different treatment preferences of different clinical practices.

Another factor driving up the charges for medical care is the fear of malpractice litigation. This argument must be couched in the context of fear, because the costs involved include more than passing on the costs of the insurance premiums, which are high. Physicians practice *defensive medicine,* which means performing all procedures the patient may believe would be helpful, and ordering additional tests during diagnosis in order to increase the statistical probability of being correct. These may seem at first blush to be appropriate actions, but often they do not change outcomes that would have occurred in their absence.

Despite the growing concern about health expenditure increases, there is little indication that the nation is somehow suffering severely as a result. It cannot be stated with certainty that health care expenditures are too high compared to other purposes for which the United States spends its gross national product (GNP). There is a growing recognition, however, that spending ever-increasing sums on health care is restricting other uses of those resources. This is certainly the case for the federal government, and the pinch is being felt in the private sector as well. In 1989, employers averaged $2,748 per employee in payments for health benefits. In 1987 and 1988, the costs of health benefits rose 18.6 and 16.7 percent, respectively (*HealthWeek* 1990a).

During the past ten years, insurance carriers have had to pay more attention to total health care costs. Employers have objected to the expenses of higher insurance premiums as a cost of labor. After some hard bargaining by labor, many large employers have accepted most of the burden for paying those premiums, and the premiums increased far too rapidly. As a percentage of total employee compensation, employer contributions for health insurance and Medicare increased from 1.5 percent in 1964 to 4.25 percent in 1983. As a result, the employers began demanding that insurance companies contain their costs. Increases in premiums, however, continue to pose problems for employers. The average insurance premium rose another 20.5 percent in 1989, a trend that affected nearly every employer in the nation (Associated Press 1990). As the demand continued for lower-cost insurance, large employers have begun opting for self-insurance. They collect and set aside the premiums and pay claims themselves, using a carrier only as a management firm. There have been other new competitors as well, which is the basis for the second reason insurance companies are paying more attention to levels of health care expenditures— they must be able to compete based on the price of their insurance products.

I have already described the actions of the federal government to contain hospital and physician expenditures. The Medicare trust fund, the source of revenue for paying Medicare bills, is likely to incur annual and eventually total deficits if expenditures are not controlled (Crozier 1984, 115). The picture for Medicaid is no brighter. The program is under constant fiscal pressure by the federal government (its share of the program has been reduced by 4 percent since 1981) and by state governments (this is especially true in those states having difficulty balancing their budgets, a constitutional requirement for all but Vermont). Government is in a position to exert direct pressure on the health care delivery system to contain costs, and the policies of the past twenty years have done so through regulation, planning requirements, peer review, the encouragement of competition, and direct cost-containment policies.

Conclusion

Recent increases in health expenditures, even after a myriad of policies have been adopted to contain costs, are a sign that more fundamental reform of the delivery and financing of health care will be needed if we are to at least stabilize expenditures. Some would argue that the health care delivery system in the United States is in crisis because of the costs and problems in access for the uninsured. Until a problem is recognized as a concern among the majority of citizens, however, and in particular by powerful interest groups, it will not be viewed by those in political office as a crisis. The operative questions, then, are: Have increases in health care expenditures become a serious problem for powerful interests? and Is there political will to address that problem?

The answer is that we are rapidly approaching the point at which an affirmative response will be accurate. A flurry of activity began in 1991, with a variety of interest groups, including the American Medical Association and the American Hospital Association, developing and promoting plans for a national system to deliver and finance health care. Several major proposals were introduced into congressional deliberations, from both political parties. Cost escalation in the Medicare and Medicaid programs precipitated calls for reforms that would lower the cost of health care. The costs of health care for individual consumers, however, have not risen enough to generate popular support for policies that might threaten access or quality, as perceived by individuals who are pleased with the quality of care they receive. As the costs of health insurance premiums continue to increase and as those increases are passed on to employers, we can expect greater pressures to contain health care expenditures. When the call for reform reaches the level of concern, which will mean voter pressure combined with pressure from interest groups, we can expect action.

The debate about the next step to contain costs has begun and is merged with the debate about how to expand access by providing health insurance benefits to those currently uninsured. Members of the issue network are now quite active in providing further analysis of costs and suggestions for policies that might address this concern. By the time political will has been mobilized and the nation is ready to act, there should be options available. Some of those options may have already been tested at the level of state government, such as health care rationing to meet a fixed budget, currently under way in Oregon. That state's plan has generated considerable debate among researchers and policymakers concerning the efficacy of rationing health care in programs serving the poor and uninsured. Some argue that government ought not engage in rationing services until the health care delivery system has been made as efficient as possible (Brown 1991), while others argue that there is a need to turn to rationing now (Callahan 1990). Oregon's timing may not be correct, and the solution advocated by decision makers in that state to ration services provided through Medicaid may not be the best means of achieving universal access while simultaneously containing expenditures. The visibility of the Oregon efforts, however, have triggered serious consideration of rationing among members of the issue network and more widespread concern among health consumers. As consumers begin to demand more significant changes, we can expect policy entrepreneurs to push forward with the suggestions offered by the analysts in the issue network.

Although it is difficult at this time to say exactly what the policy strategy will be, it is possible to look to recent and ongoing major initiatives as building blocks of an aggressive policy of cost containment. The next chapter will do so, with examinations of health planning, prospective payment, and resource-based relative-value scales.

4

. . .

Health Care
Cost-Containment Policies

For what may seem to health care providers to be an eternity, but what is actually a history of less than twenty years, the federal government has engaged in concerted efforts to restrain the growth in health care expenditures, particularly those expenditures financed through the Medicare program. At times the resulting policies have affected all sources of payment because they were aimed at controlling the supply of health care services. At other times they have focused on the demand for health by constraining payments, such as limiting hospital payments as incentives to discharge patients more quickly. Even the more narrowly construed policies, however, have broader implications. Medicare is a predominant payer for many providers and will therefore influence their behavior if certain conditions are set as prerequisites for receiving Medicare payment. Other payers will often follow Medicare's lead if a new payment scheme is successful in constraining expenditures. Government policies help determine how health care is financed and therefore influence total expenditures.

This is not to argue, however, that policies and practices of other providers are not important in determining the means and amounts of payment. Large insurance companies and large self-insured corporations determine their own payment policies, which health care providers accept because those companies represent a significant share of the revenue for providers. State governments can also influence health care financing policy, particularly through their actions in the Medicaid program. As is the case with large insurers and corporations, states can exert some influence because of the percent of health care clients their beneficiaries represent. This is especially true for Medicaid clients in long-term care facilities; in many nursing homes a majority of the clients may be Medicaid recipients. State Medicaid programs have somewhat less leverage with physicians because their beneficiaries will represent a small percentage of total income to physicians. In fact, many physicians decline to treat any Medicaid clients.

In this chapter, I will focus on the major federal government cost-containment efforts since 1975. The discussion will include an analysis of the political motivations for certain policies and an explanation of their enactment consistent with the framework for policy development presented in chapters 1 and 2. As will be evident, we can learn a great deal about the general policy propensities of government by focusing on specific policies. A less extensive discussion of private sector and state government initiatives will be included. Finally, in the concluding section I will discuss the general prospects for success in the battle to constrain health care expenditure increases.

Health Planning to Control Supply

By the 1970s, evidence analyzed by health services researchers showed conclusively that the additional supply of health care facilities actually increased expenditures, contrary to conventional economic wisdom that increased supply will result in lower prices because of increased competition. In the case of health care, supply seems to generate demand, resulting in an increase in aggregate expenditures. Data available at the time indicated that for every million dollars in capital expansion, $350,000 to $400,000 was added to annual operating expenses (Somers 1969). When Congress was considering extending such programs as the Hill-Burton construction grants for health facilities and comprehensive health planning, the analytical conclusion being offered through the issue network was that unneeded health care facilities were causing increases in health expenditures. Therefore, it seemed logical to enact a policy that would allow only *needed* facilities to be built. Need for facilities could be determined through a planning process, and final decisions would include some input from the citizens of the community.

The National Health Planning and Resources Development Act of 1974 (Public Law 93-641) became law on 4 January 1975. The act marked the transition from access to cost containment as the principal theme in federal health policy. Advocates for both of these objectives supported health planning, but the program's purposes quickly became defined solely in terms of containing health care expenditures. Seen through that prism, the program was judged a failure and was terminated in 1986. The life history of this program offers important lessons both in how health policies are developed and in the enormous difficulties inherent in attempting to control health care expenditures.

THE DEVELOPMENT OF HEALTH PLANNING

During the early 1970s the issue network in health policy had worked to develop an acceptable proposal for national health insurance. If a national system were to be enacted, there seemed to be a need to rationalize the delivery of health care. Without that preliminary action, a system that provided unlimited access to all types of health care for all citizens could be driven to bankruptcy. The health planning legislation drafted in the early 1970s, supported by Kennedy and Javits in the Senate and Rogers and Staggers in the House, created a network of administrative agencies through which a new program of national health insurance could be administered. These agencies would both plan for a rational delivery system and prepare for the administration of such a program.

The legislation enacted in 1975 embodied two characteristics that were the by-products of the political climate of the times, both of which were to cause problems later. First, during the heyday of the Great Society programs of the 1960s, an attitude developed among national government officials that they knew better than states and localities how to design effective social policies. Autonomous health systems agencies were created that were not the creatures of state governments but instead separately constituted organizations whose jurisdiction could cross state boundaries or any other political demarcations. This strategy quickly became a political football in many states where governors were displeased with their inability to control the new health systems agencies (HSAs). Second, this new program was part of an ongoing effort to increase citizen participation in government decision making. As a consequence, at least 50 percent of the board for each HSA had to be consumers, persons not employed in the health care industry. This requirement created controversy for the program because it made the judgments of the HSAs suspect in the eyes of experts while it created organizations easily swayed by expert testimony.

Compromises were struck in 1974 that mollified the opposition to the health planning legislation, overcoming the objections of the most powerful professional interest groups. For example, the American Hospital Association objected to suggestions that existing health care facilities be subject to review to determine whether or not they were appropriate for the community's needs. Thanks to a compromise making the findings of any such reviews advisory only, HSAs lacked any power to affect existing situations of oversupply in communities. Even this minimal power of review and advice was effectively eliminated because no funds were ever appropriated for that purpose. To satisfy state governments that the new program was not a threat to their authority, governors were given the power to review appeals from providers disappointed with HSA decisions. Finally, provisions for rate review and approval of doctor and hospital charges were removed from early drafts of the legislation. The combination of compromises concerning appropriateness review, certificate-of-need (CON) reviews (placing final approval powers under the governor), and the removal of rate regulation made the planning process ineffective as a cost-containment strategy.

The American Medical Association (AMA) opposed the 1974 legislation, testifying that it would make health care a public utility. Although this argument did not defeat the program in Congress, the AMA's opposition was responsible at least in part for omitting provisions that would have applied CON requirements to equipment in doctors' offices and provisions mandating that states set rates of reimbursement for medical procedures. The American Hospital Association (AHA) also opposed mandatory rate-setting, as well as early provisions in the legislation that would have required closing facilities determined to be in excess of community need.

The AHA did not, however, oppose health planning in principle, and the Federation of American Hospitals (the for-profit counterpart to the AHA) endorsed health planning. Existing hospitals actually stood to benefit from health planning, absent any provisions to reduce current supply. Any new competitors would be required to undergo review and to prove the need for additional hospital beds in the community. Given the state of affairs of the past twenty years, proving need for additional beds is difficult at best. Further, current providers in the community are afforded the opportunity to testify against the need for new facilities, an argument that they usually present persuasively. The Nixon administration supported health planning, favoring its own suggestions over the bill introduced by members of Congress. The health insurance industry was strongly supportive as was the American Health Planning Association (AHPA).

The common sentiment of interest groups in the issue network was in favor of health planning, and analysts in the network provided the ammunition to support the efficacy of planning. The key to success in obtaining the program, though, was the support of influential policy entrepreneurs in Congress, Senator Kennedy and Representative Rogers in particular. In their vision, particularly for Senator Kennedy and other Senate supporters (such as Senator Javits of New York), this legislation was intended first to rationalize health care delivery, then to provide administrative support to health planning. A consequence of making the system more rational would be constraining increases in expenditures because of oversupply, but the original intent was not that the planning program be a major cost-containment effort: "The planning program was not intended to be a major cost containment device, and it lacks the authority needed to control expenditures" (Committee on Health Planning Goals and Standards 1981, 7). The planning program was based on an assumption that it would provide a means of integrating community participation with the tools of planning, to both restrain unnecessary growth in the health care delivery system and establish a system responsive to the health care needs of communities. The program was enacted at a time when national health insurance was thought to be just around the corner and steps were needed to prepare for its inevitability.

THE PROGRAM IN TROUBLE

During the early 1970s, health planning was viewed as a means of introducing data analysis into public decisions concerning permitting the expansion of health care facilities. Health care expenditures were controlled more directly as one commodity falling under the rules and constraints of the Economic Stabilization Program. When that program ended, though, health care costs exploded, and public officials turned to health planning and CON as the best existing option for cost containment. This meant a shift in focus for the program to a purpose for which it was not designed. True, the program was intended to curb expenditures related to expansion of health care facilities, but those costs represented only a portion of all health care expenditures. Even in its modest objectives to contain costs, the program was drawn narrowly. Some of the compromises included in the 1974 legislation would now cause severe problems in implementation.

For example, state governments could overturn the recommendations of local health system agencies (HSAs), and many did so. An official of the Department of Health, Education, and Welfare (HEW) admitted in testimony to Congress in 1978 that specific instances of such actions occurred in Ohio and Massachusetts. The original provisions of the legislation designed to provide powers to lower expenditures by removing unnecessary facilities and by regulating capital expansion throughout the system were removed, leaving very little to regulate.

The success of this program in controlling costs rested on the use of CON to decrease spending on unnecessary facilities. The AHPA presented evidence of such savings in 1979, of $2.3 billion to $3.5 billion, or eight dollars for every one dollar spent (Hearings before the Subcommittee on Health and the Environment, 1979). Their survey of HSAs also found that 3,700 proposed hospital beds were disapproved. Among skilled nursing homes and intermediate care facilities, 114,000 new beds were proposed (85,000 officially); 49,000 did not get approved (20,000 were officially denied). They claimed the resulting savings in operating costs would exceed $10 billion in the 1980s.

Members of particular HSAs testifying in those same hearings cited specific examples of the effectiveness of the CON process; in Birmingham, Alabama, a new 144-bed hospital was denied because it was within 10 minutes driving time of two existing hospitals, and a new open-heart surgery proposal was rejected because there was already excess capacity in the region. Similar findings from a study commissioned by the Health Insurance Association of America (HIAA) were cited by the assistant secretary of Health and Human Services (HHS, formerly HEW) in Senate hearings in 1979: "Information obtained from 29 of the 50 states by HIAA indicates that CON disapprovals totalled $700 million against approvals of $3.9 billion" (Hearings before the Subcommittee on Health and Scientific Research 1979, 133).

The body of evidence just presented would seem to be quite persuasive. Those presenting the data, however, were advocates of health planning. By the later 1970s, the composition of the issue network in health issues had changed somewhat, and critics of health planning were included who could, and did, present evidence critical of the program. For example, the General Accounting Office (GAO, created by Congress to provide independent analysis) described four types of errors in the AHPA calculations: (1) including projects initially disapproved, then later approved; (2) including projects built despite being disapproved; (3) including projects withdrawn because of an inability to acquire debt financing; and (4) multiple counting of projects disapproved each time they were disapproved (Eastaugh 1987).

Economists have been particularly critical of CON, presenting evidence that it saves very little when compared to the billions spent for health care. A study of the effectiveness of CON as used in some states through 1975 concluded that restricting growth in new hospital beds would merely induce other expenses (Sloan and Steinwald 1980). Although bed growth may be reduced, more assets may be devoted to each remaining bed, increasing aggregate costs (Salkever and Bice 1976).

When a CON process was initially required by federal statute, many hospital capital development programs were already under way. Continued operating expense increases would be experienced, then, as those projects were completed. Savings from controlling current capital development would not be realized until some time in the future. Some scholarly literature supported the conclusion that CON generated cost savings that were not apparent until several years after it was adopted (Davis 1982). A study of Massachusetts's efforts over a more expanded period of time revealed that several years after enactment of initial legislation it became effective because of a change in personnel administering the program. The results of that change would not appear in aggregate data until another lag occurred so that capital projects already in the pipeline would be completed. This finding formed the basis of criticism of earlier studies showing no effect of CON: "At this juncture, therefore, little systematic information on the ultimate outcome of mature certificate-of-need programs in limiting hospital capital expenditure has been developed" (Howell 1984, 608). During debates about the adequacy of health planning and CON, though, only early evidence was available. Further, there were respected scholars in the issue network arguing that CON made little difference as a cost-containment device.

Interest groups debated its effectiveness during the 1970s and into the 1980s, with, as expected, the AHPA strongly endorsing the program and the AMA continuing to oppose it. Hospital groups were somewhat neutral during the debates, perhaps because they had learned how to "game" the system by persuading local consumers to accede to hospital requests for expansion (Mueller and Comer 1983). Other groups also provided support for the program (the insurance industry and big business), and state governors continued to press for greater state level involvement (Iglehart 1975b).

Principal support for the program during its midlife came from entrepreneurs in Congress. Representative Waxman, as chair of the House Subcommittee on Health of the Energy and Commerce Committee, was especially supportive throughout the program's history, and some observers give him most of the credit for keeping the program alive and well into the 1980s.

Throughout the existence of this program, debates combined ideological perspectives with analysis based on empirical data. There were strong proponents who viewed attacks on the huge, monolithic health care industry as a crusade, and there were opponents who viewed any government regulation as inherently counterproductive. Scholars attempted to contribute to the debates with analysis of expenditure data, but interpreting the data proved difficult and

73

open to criticism regardless of the conclusions drawn. In such a policy environment, programs are ripe for attack when the climate of the times and/or the composition of the issue network change(s).

HEALTH PLANNING DIES

The federal health planning program sputtered during the early 1980s, ending in 1986. Changes in the policy environment and the issue network contributed to the death of this program. The beginning of the end for this program was the inauguration of Ronald Reagan as president in 1981.

The 1980 election signaled changes in the policy environment toward a reduction of federal government activity in domestic policy issues, and toward an acceleration of deregulation throughout the domestic economy. Three specific changes in the environment for health policies are of special note (Mueller 1988a). The first was a new system of paying hospitals for Medicare clients, the prospective payment system (PPS), enacted in 1983. The PPS is now the reigning tool for controlling expenditures for hospital care, usurping the role of health planning for that purpose. Since cost containment continued as the dominant theme in the 1980s, health planning became vulnerable as an unnecessary program.

The second change was the emergence of the federal budget as the single most important concern in each session of Congress. As deficits mounted during the 1980s, Congress increasingly looked for means of reducing federal spending. Under those circumstances all federal programs have been under increased pressure to prove their worth, and health planning was especially vulnerable. The third change was in the partisan alignment in the Congress, with a Republican majority in the Senate until 1987 and a larger percentage of Republicans in the House. This constituted a change in the issue network but also a change in the policy environment. The turnover signaled a mood change in the electorate, to which all members of Congress were responsive. Therefore, policy arguments that incorporated themes of reducing government interference and allowed for more private sector competition carried favor. These arguments were used against health planning.

Changes in the issue network also accounted for the demise of the health planning program. The most obvious among them was the change in presidential administrations. Along with that change, the influence of the Office of Management and Budget (OMB) in health policy matters increased after 1981. There were two reasons for this: the budget crisis made the role of budget offi-

74

cers more all-encompassing across all spending programs, and the Reagan administration increased the power of the OMB in reviewing the activities of all federal agencies (Mueller 1988). The AHA changed its position from lukewarm support of the program to strong opposition in 1985, declaring the program to be too inflexible. Although Representative Waxman continued to be a strong supporter of the program, his influence was weakened somewhat by the change in the composition of his subcommittee from 12–5 in favor of the Democrats to 14–9, and in the full committee from 27–15 to 25–17. Finally, the AMA made the demise of health planning a high priority in 1985, seeing its vulnerability as an opportunity for a legislative victory.

The beginning of the end for this program came in 1981, when Congress included in budget legislation a provision allowing states to dismantle local health systems agencies. As those agencies began to phase out, hospitals returned to earlier tendencies to build new additions and add expensive equipment (Demkovich 1983). The influence of medical lobbies in state governments contributed to quick actions in several states to dismantle HSAs (Mueller and Comer 1991).

The prospects for continuing this program were poor each year beginning in 1981, since the presidential budget proposal consistently recommended terminating all funding. During 1985, opponents of the program used effectively the popular policy themes of deregulation and decentralization to argue for terminating the program. The final vote to reauthorize this program was 22–20 against in Waxman's subcommittee, effectively killing health planning. All of the factors discussed above were instrumental, and the final blow was a result of last-minute vote switching in the subcommittee (Mueller 1988a).

THE LEGACY OF HEALTH PLANNING

Federal involvement in health planning included the expectation of containing health care expenditures and ended because that expectation was not met. State and local commitments to health planning, however, have not evaporated, and the federally funded program contributed to expanding the issue network in health policy to include informed consumers. As we move toward policies to reshape health care delivery and finance, we may witness a resurgence of federal interest in health planning.

Not all state governments have given up on health planning as a tool to constrain growth in health expenditures. The certificate-of-need program, the cornerstone of cost containment through planning, was retained by thirty-eight states after Congress repealed the national law requiring those programs. Apparently those states continue to be persuaded by the evidence that planning can save health care expenditures by denying capital growth of health care facilities and equipment. In 1992 eight additional states were considering adopting CON laws. The targets of CON laws may not always be hospitals, the subject of the debates and legislation in the 1970s. Instead, the concerns of the 1990s are nursing homes, psychiatric facilities, and expensive equipment. The owners of those facilities are less powerful than hospitals in influencing policies and less capable of altering policies during implementation. The success of state CON laws is a function of the changes in the issue network given the foci of those laws.

States use health planning in ways other than the review of petitions to add capital expenditures. Over thirty-five states have established state offices of rural health, many of which use the methods of health planning (such as needs assessment and consideration of alternative strategies for delivering services) to provide assistance to medical care providers and rural communities. Oregon's Office of Rural Health provides assistance to hospitals to identify the strengths and weaknesses of their institutions, and Florida's health department completed a study of the problems of rural hospitals (Mueller 1988c). State health programs, such as HIV/AIDS education and prevention efforts, rely on planning to forecast future needs and effectively target limited resources. State mental health planning grants from the federal government fund the development of comprehensive mental health plans.

The legacy of the federally funded effort in health planning includes a new awareness among consumers of their influence in decisions about how health care will be financed and delivered. Before the health planning program and the use of health systems agencies, medical providers dominated all decisions—national, state, and local—concerning health care finance and delivery. As HSAS gained experience in dealing with questions of capital and with writing health plans for localities and states, the power of the medical provider diminished: "The simple repetition of the HSAS' regulatory circus, year after year in every community, stripped the medical profession of its authority over medical politics" (Morone 1990a, 318). The new players in the issue network, local consumers, faded into the woodwork when HSAS disbanded. By the late 1970s, over 9,000 consumers and providers served on HSAS, and an additional 35,000 citizens served on committees created by HSAS. Statewide health coordinating councils, created in compliance with the federal law, included nearly 1,800 consumers. Most of these new participants in health policy decision making remain active in their states and localities (Morone, 1990a). These individuals and many community associations of active consumers (such as business coalitions, public interest groups, and local foundations) are an effective balance to the traditional concerns of medical care providers.

Local activists in health planning could form the nucleus of a renewed effort to incorporate health planning into national health policy. The terms may be changed to more palatable descriptions such as "integration of services," or "coordination of activities," or "information analysis," but the concepts and thrusts will be similar to the original intentions of the 1974 legislation. The idea that planning could continue at the local level and even see a renewal of use starting with community planning was foreseen by Dr. John Ball from the American College of Physicians in his 1982 testimony on repealing the program: "There is a need for health planning; that is, a structure and process for determining primarily at the local level what health services are wanted and will be encouraged in each community" (Subcommittee on Health and the Environment 1982, 171). Ball accurately described the planning in place today in many states and localities, and his statement provides the reasoning for believing we will once again turn to such a scheme as a national effort.

Further evidence of the need for, and benefits of, planning can be found in the experiences of other nations. Other nations use the methods of health planning to restrict the supply of advanced medical technology, which in turn helps them keep the costs of health care below those experienced in the United States (Grogan 1992). As the debate over how to reform the health care system in this country continues, we should expect arguments for reintroducing national health planning. In fact, as early as 1988 there were initial rumblings in Congress that health planning should again be supported by the federal government (Sorian 1988). As is often the case in public policy, what goes around comes around.

CONCLUDING COMMENTS ABOUT PLANNING

This description of health planning as a federal policy activity has served to illustrate two themes of this book. First, the evolution of health policy from emphasizing access to a concern for cost containment was evident in how this program was perceived and evaluated. Second, the importance of changes in the policy environment and issue network was evident in the demise of this program.

Is planning a bad idea? The program's demise was more a result of political changes than of thorough analysis of the efficacy of planning. As new issues have surfaced in recent years, particularly in access to services, health planning activities are beginning to resume an important role in health policy. Planning, however, is not seen as a panacea for reducing or containing health expenditures. Instead, the activities that characterize planning, (that is, assessing the availability and coordination of health care services), are being conducted for the purposes of assuring access to appropriate services. Planning will become even more important should the nation once again begin a march toward a national system.

Hospital Payment Policies

Health planning, through the power of CON review, was a tool to contain hospital costs. However, hospital charges continued to increase throughout the 1970s. With CON as a tool to control capital expenditures by hospitals, other policies have focused on the operating expenses by establishing some form of control over hospital charges. There are three basic approaches to controlling hospital charges. First, charges for specific services can be tightly regulated, with specific fee schedules. This action is undertaken primarily by state governments and has met with mixed results. Second, a more general fee schedule can be established that, rather than tightly regulating charges made by individual hospitals, establishes a prospective payment for general categories of treatment that will be applied to all hospitals. This is the approach taken by the federal government since 1983 and the enactment of the prospective payment system (PPS) based on diagnosis-related groups (DRGs). Third, a system could be created that establishes "global budgets" for hospitals that set maximum total annual revenues for the hospitals, which include all services offered by any particular hospital during a budget year. This has been suggested as a mechanism that could contain hospital expenditures, based on its use in other countries.

DIRECT REGULATION

A few states have used a direct regulatory approach to determine how much hospitals would be reimbursed. A variety of methods have been used, including limiting payments to a fixed percentage of hospital charges, reimbursing only what the state determines is a "reasonable" amount for a given service, and determining in advance total expenditures to be paid to hospitals for the coming year. The last method has been tried only on an experimental basis; the first two have been used frequently.

Four states (New Jersey, Maryland, Massachusetts, and New York) pioneered prospective payment, though not based on diagnosis-related groups, in the early 1970s. Their programs were moderately successful in containing expenditures (Gaus and Hellinger 1976). Although some studies have given evidence of the cost-effectiveness of state regulation programs (Hadley and Schwartz 1989), overall the success of these programs has been mixed. They are effective in reducing short-term hospital expenses, restraining them to levels similar to increases in general health care inflation. Unless they address the underlying causes of expenditure increases, however, including the manner in which medicine is practiced, they will not provide long-term success in containing expenditures.

With the exception of price controls as part of the Economic Stabilization Program of the early 1970s during the Nixon presidency, the national government has not used a similar regulatory approach. President Carter proposed in 1979 that hospital fees be regulated by the federal government. That proposal suffered legislative defeat after the hospital industry offered to restrain cost increases voluntarily. Congress indicated a willingness to let the private sector resolve the cost problem on its own, consistent with the American preference to minimize government interference in the private marketplace. Initially the voluntary effort seemed successful, but within two years hospital expenditures were again increasing rapidly.

During these same years the issue network in health care in the national government had changed, as indicated in the previous discussion of health planning. Ronald Reagan assumed the presidency in 1981, bringing with him an ideology opposed to covert government regulation and favoring reductions in federal commitments to social programs. Partisan leadership in the U.S. Senate changed in 1981 from the Democrats to the Republicans, and the chair of the Labor and Human Resources Committee passed from Edward Kennedy to Orrin Hatch. The perspective of these new players (including members of the Reagan administration) was that if competition was introduced into the health care delivery system, costs would be controlled. Incentives could be used to influence hospital administrators to control their costs and thereby control charges.

In addition to changes in the issue network, the general political climate in Congress changed in the early 1980s. The politics of federal budgeting have resulted in searches for any possible savings in federal spending. The savings are measured in terms of dollars not spent that would have been spent were it not for legislative decisions. Thus, the savings are from anticipated spending, not current spending. As the most rapidly increasing expenditures in anyone's budget, including that of the federal government, health expenditures are favorite targets for such policy choices. Hospital expenditures have long represented the largest share of Medicare expenditures, so hospital-cost containment assumed a heightened importance with the dawn of budgetary politics.

By 1982, members of Congress and the administration were convinced that the voluntary effort to contain hospital expenditures was a failure. Congress used the Tax Equity and Fiscal Responsibility Act of 1982 (TEFRA) as the legislative vehicle to reduce, over three years, reimbursement for hospitals by $5 billion and to require from the Department of Health and Human Services (DHHS) a new system for reimbursement that would determine amounts prospectively (Iglehart 1982b). This approach should encourage providers to reduce costs below preset levels in order to increase profit, or return on investment. At the same time, the important political objective of being able to budget Medicare expenses would be accomplished. Rather than promising to pay audited costs plus a margin, reimbursement can be determined in advance and set to stay within the limits desired by Congress.

At the time DHHS was required to develop a scheme for prospective payment of hospitals, a system was being tried in New Jersey funded as a demonstration grant by DHHS. Researchers at Yale University helped develop a system to classify hospital admissions for the purpose of reimbursement. The classifications are based on the primary and secondary medical diagnoses of the patients upon admission. The program there had begun in 1978, and by 1982 it was viewed enthusiastically by state officials in New Jersey and federal officials in DHHS (Iglehart 1982a).

DETERMINATION OF PAYMENT UNDER PPS

In amendments to the Social Security Act, Congress adopted the prospective payment system in 1983 as the means of paying hospitals for treating Medicare patients. Since 1983 legislative debate about Medicare payment of hospitals has centered on technical adjustments to the PPS and allowable rate increases in the basic calculation of rates. In order to understand the nature of those debates it is necessary to review briefly the technical basis for calculating payment under the new system.

Payment is based on the nature of the service rendered, which is categorized as one of 467 diagnosis-related groups (DRGs). The principal contribution of the Yale researchers assisting in the New Jersey demonstration was the creation of 383 diagnostic categories, later increased to 467, which are derived from the

23 major diagnostic categories in the International Classification of Diseases. In this scheme, each major diagnostic category is divided into principal diagnoses, which are in turn divided into specific diagnosis-related groups; the final DRG is a "residual" category, accounting for diagnoses not included in the others. The resulting DRGs account for all Medicare discharges in a given year.

After the DRGs are established, the next step is to calculate reimbursement rates for each DRG. During the first four years of PPS, the rates were a blend of calculations based on the previous charges of individual hospitals and the national average. Since 1988 a single national average has been used. The base charge, from which adjustments are made based on the DRG and other considerations, is the average total charge for Medicare inpatient hospital stays. The following criteria are used to adjust the rate by multiplying average hospital charges by the following weighting factors:

1. the average length of stay associated with a particular DRG;
2. a case mix index, which represents the service intensity associated with particular DRGs;
3. the prevailing wage rates in the region;
4. the number of medical school residents working in the hospital;
5. the number of poor (Medicaid and charity) patients as a percentage of all patients.

The calculation of the PPS rate is displayed in Figure 4.1. Separate rates were calculated from 1983 through 1995 for urban and rural hospitals. Additional adjustments can be made if particular cases treated by the hospital are classified as outliers, meaning that either the patient has stayed well beyond the average number of days and/or the actual charges for that patient's care far exceed the reimbursement allowed under PPS.

Each year Congress determines the change from the previous year that will be allowed in the base rate used in calculating PPS reimbursements. The Prospective Payment Review Commission (PROPAC) was created by Congress to provide recommendations for the annual changes, as well as analysis and advice concerning other issues related to the new payment system. Commission members are appointed by the president, chosen to represent various interest groups as well as provide technical expertise. Their input is intended to "sanitize" the rate-setting process by providing apolitical recommendations to Congress, based on their independent analysis rather than partisan sentiment. In considering adjustments to the annual rates, the commission considers such factors as the costs of new technologies and medicines, improvements in hospi-

81

```
P = AC • DRG • UC • WI • TH + OUT
Payment = Average Cost for Hospital Admission
              * Weighting based on Diagnosis-Related Groups
              * Weighting based on Uncompensated Care
              * Weighting for Wage Index
              * Weighting for Teaching Hospitals
              + Allowance for outlier
```

Figure 4.1 Calculation of prospective payment for hospitals (PPS rate).

tal productivity, changes in wages, and changes in general hospital costs. PRO-PAC also examines other issues in the payment system, such as the appropriateness of eliminating the separate distinction for rural hospitals, basing outlier payments on different criteria, and changing the adjustments for the costs of medical education. Most recently, PROPAC has provided input related to including the costs of capital in PPS calculations. In short, PROPAC and its staff have become important and influential members of the issue network dealing with hospital payment policies.

The secretary of Health and Human Services also recommends annual rate changes to Congress, and his or her recommendations are those of the administration, after the OMB has approved them for submission to Congress. The concern about the federal budget deficit drives the administration's recommendations. The rates can be adjusted to lower projected hospital expenditures and thereby claim budget savings. In many years since 1983, the rate has been set as a *reduction* after adjusting for the costs of goods and services purchased by hospitals, called the "market basket." In fiscal years 1988 and 1989, for example, the rates were increased by market basket minus varying percentages for urban, rural, and inner-city hospitals. An implicit promise from Congress to providers was that after the first few years of fine tuning in the PPS, increases would be equal to the market basket, but two political debates have intervened. First, during the early years of PPS, hospitals continue to earn high profits on Medicare patients (Iglehart 1986), so Congress approved recommendations that "ratcheted down" the reimbursement rates. Second, continued pressure to reduce federal deficits has forced Congress to look for ways to reduce budget commitments to Medicare. As the one part of that program in which expenditures can be controlled directly, the PPS has been used to achieve these budget objectives.

USING PPS TO ACHIEVE NONPAYMENT POLICY OBJECTIVES

During the 1980s, Medicare payments policies were the major game in town for federal health policy. Therefore, the decisions involving the payment system were often decisions to assure access or quality. A major debate during the 1980s concerned whether or not the reimbursement provided rural hospitals was sufficient to assure that these hospitals could afford to continue providing services to Medicare patients. This concern will be given more attention in the next chapter as an issue in access for rural citizens, but it deserves mention here as an issue in Medicare payment policies.

When the PPS was enacted in 1983, the data available to Congress demonstrated a difference in hospital inpatient charges between urban and rural facilities, with the latter charging far less. Even after examining reasons for the differences related to the types of patients seen and types of care provided, differences remained between urban and rural charges. The new payment system created different rates for urban and rural hospitals, based on their historical differences in charges. That differential was subsequently blamed for the fiscal woes that many rural hospitals confronted. By the end of the 1980s, Congress agreed that the differential was a mistake, and it was scheduled for elimination by 1995.

During the years of the urban-rural differential payment scheme, Congress created special categories of rural hospitals in an effort to provide higher reimbursement to those rural hospitals with higher costs and those that were essential to certain communities. The former were designated as rural referral centers, because they received patients from other rural facilities, much the same as larger urban hospitals. Referral centers have been reimbursed at the urban rate. Essential hospitals are designated as "sole community providers," and they have been reimbursed based on their own historical charges rather than on an average of all hospitals. The most recent change in reimbursement was to create two new categories of rural hospitals, essential access care hospitals, and primary care hospitals. This step was taken in 1991 and will be discussed in the next chapter.

The payment system is also adjusted to achieve other policy objectives. For example, Congress wants to continue providing support for teaching activities and uses an adjustment factor in the PPS (see figure 4.1) to pay a little more to hospitals with teaching programs. Similarly, additional payments are given to hospitals that serve a disproportionate number of patients unable to pay their bills or hospitals with a disproportionate number of Medicaid patients.

Given the importance of deficit reduction through changes in hospital payment and the opportunity to affect hospital behavior through changes in the formulas, actors in the issue network wanting to influence policy have focused on the PPS. Hospitals have certainly been active lobbyists in attempting to maximize their return under the rules of the formula. Presidential administrations have used the PPS as a means of achieving budget savings, and members of Congress have used it to respond to the demands of their constituencies. During the first several years of the program, members of Congress with rural constituencies were especially vocal. By the beginning of the 1990s, members with central city districts, where hospitals are also experiencing economic difficulties, became equally vocal.

This particular policy issue provides an excellent opportunity to describe the importance of the analysis provided by some members of the issue network. Foremost among those persons are the staff and members of PROPAC, whose technical analysis and recommendations provide the grist for annual policy debates about changing the reimbursement rate. Other researchers have provided analysis related to issues involving rural hospitals, technical adjustments to the payment for teaching hospitals, and technical changes in the calculations used in the formula. Finally, technical analysis is used to establish the base (hospital "market basket" costs) from which the calculations are made and to suggest changes to update, or "rebase," that formula.

The debate concerning hospital reimbursement hinges on definitions and proofs of fair payment. This requires information concerning actual costs of providing services, reasonable rates of return on investment, and linkages between charges and specific services. Analysts from PROPAC are joined by scholars and analysts working for particular interest groups in providing technical analysis. This can be expected to continue until a more comprehensive payment system, such as global budgeting, might replace PPS as the federal method of choice.

THE EFFECTIVENESS OF PPS

Three questions can be asked about the effectiveness of the PPS. The first is, Is the basis for calculating rates the best we can devise? Although the DRG-based formulas used in the system are statistically powerful, they are based on analysis that still does not account for all the actual variation in hospital costs. Significant differences in costs still exist within single DRGs. Patients admitted with identical DRGs may have different levels of severity, e.g., some are at greater risk from higher and more persistent fevers, and so on. Patients in the same DRG therefore require varying resources during the hospital stay. Several researchers have been working to incorporate severity of illness measures into the DRG calculations, and the Health Care Finance Administration (HCFA), which administers the Medicare program, is continuing to sponsor such research in hopes of improving the PPS calculations.

Theoretically, if the PPS is based on averages, even when experience varies within any particular DRG, hospitals will still, in the long run, receive fair reimbursement. When the number of cases within DRGs is low, however, variation can result in payments that either underpay or overpay, as a percentage of actual expenses. Small rural hospitals are especially likely to suffer under these conditions, because Medicare patients are a large portion of their total patients, but still low in aggregate numbers. Although additional payment for outliers provides some relief from large costs, those payments are not based on 100 percent of actual costs, and in order to receive them, the case has to be extraordinarily more expensive than the average.

Since the PPS is based on statistical calculations, the variables and techniques used are important and subject to technical criticism. For example, the adjustment for teaching hospitals has been challenged as too liberal because of the regression equations used in its calculation (Thorpe 1988). Other challenges to the calculations in the PPS have focused on how outlier payments are determined, how rural referral centers are reimbursed, how sole community hospitals are classified, and how the costs of technology are built into the system. In short, work continues on fine-tuning the PPS formula. Various analysts in the issue network, based in academic institutions or think tanks, contribute their independent research and recommendations during this process. Various interest groups in the network will conduct their own analyses, offering statistical as well as political challenges to the formula. For example, the American Hospital Association (AHA) has conducted extensive analysis of the wage index used in calculating reimbursement rates and successfully argued for change in how the index is calculated and applied. Given the requirement that the system remain budget-neutral by not increasing overall expenses for Medicare hospital payments, changes are determined in part by technical analysis and in part after struggles in the political battlefield between competing groups.

The second question concerning effectiveness is Has the PPS achieved the objective of controlling public expenditures? On the face of it the answer is *yes,* since Congress can set the annual adjustment rates according to budget needs as easily as according to the analytical recommendations of the PROPAC and others. The implicit objective of the program, however, is that it would actually influence decision making by hospital officials and medical care providers such that aggregate expenses, including those passed on to payers other than Medicare, would be controlled.

In the aggregate, hospital expenditures have continued to increase dramatically in recent years. As demonstrated in figure 4.2, however, much of the recent increase has been in outpatient expenditures, which are not subject to the PPS. On the inpatient side, expenditures have also increased at a rate exceeding the one intended by the modest allowable increases in the PPS and faster than the market-basket index for hospitals. How could this be so? There are three fundamental limits of the PPS to control *aggregate* hospital expenditures. First, rates of admission to hospitals are not controlled, so increases in hospital admissions would increase expenditures even if the cost per admission is controlled (Wennberg et al. 1984). Available evidence shows that aggregate hospital admissions have declined since the implementation of the PPS, but that they have been rising again the past two years, as shown in figure 4.3.

A second explanation for increases in aggregate hospital expenditures is that the new Medicare system applies only to Medicare patients. Hospitals are still able to increase charges to other payers and realize increases in revenue, perhaps even compensating for lost revenue from the Medicare program. In fact, many hospital administrators and insurance carriers claim this has become a common practice because hospitals are shifting their costs from the tightly controlled Medicare program to the less constrained private reimbursement systems. The result is that Medicare is effective in controlling its own annual changes in expenditures for hospitalization, while the overall rate continues a more rapid pace of annual increase, as shown in figure 4.4.

The third means of increasing hospital expenditures in spite of the PPS is to diversify hospital business beyond the inpatient programs. The increase in outpatient expenditures is an indication that this has happened since 1983. Evidence of this affecting the Medicare program is scant; in fact, some have concluded that it has not happened and that the Medicare program has saved substantial sums under the PPS (Russell and Manning 1989).

The third question about the effectiveness of this program is What is the impact on the health care delivery system? The implicit aspiration of those in favor of the system, using the procompetition philosophy of the new actors in the health policy issue network, is that the PPS will result in more efficient delivery of care without any sacrifices in quality or access. In a study using data from the early years when those paid by the PPS rules could be compared with those paid

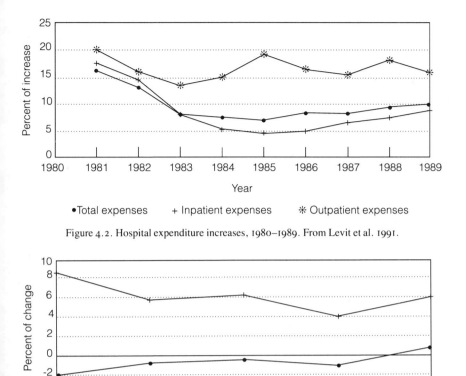

Figure 4.2. Hospital expenditure increases, 1980–1989. From Levit et al. 1991.

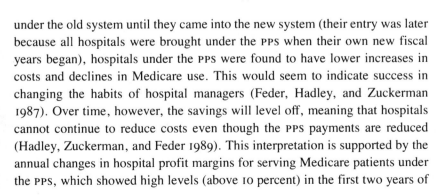

Figure 4.3. Annual change in hospital admissions and outpatient visits, 1986–1990 (est.). From Cowan et al. 1991.

under the old system until they came into the new system (their entry was later because all hospitals were brought under the PPS when their own new fiscal years began), hospitals under the PPS were found to have lower increases in costs and declines in Medicare use. This would seem to indicate success in changing the habits of hospital managers (Feder, Hadley, and Zuckerman 1987). Over time, however, the savings will level off, meaning that hospitals cannot continue to reduce costs even though the PPS payments are reduced (Hadley, Zuckerman, and Feder 1989). This interpretation is supported by the annual changes in hospital profit margins for serving Medicare patients under the PPS, which showed high levels (above 10 percent) in the first two years of

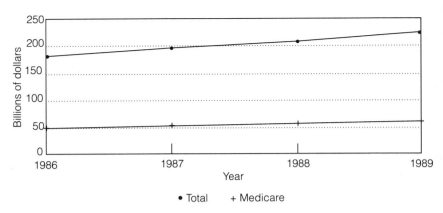

Figure 4.4. Hospital expenditures: Medicare and total, 1986–1989. From Lazenby and Letsch, 1990.

the system, but then shrank in later years into the negative range for rural hospitals. Overall margins also declined during those years to less than four percent for all hospitals (Guterman, Altman, and Young 1990).

The PPS may have unintended consequences affecting the care of Medicare patients. The system creates an incentive to discharge patients earlier than had been the case, supposedly to a more appropriate care environment. This could mean more effective use of home health care, or more frequent use of long-term care facilities that provide twenty-four-hour nursing assistance to patients. The system is not intended to discharge patients before their need ends for acute care services that can only be provided in a full-service hospital.

Issues about quality of care arise when patients are discharged from hospitals when they still need special medical attention. Unless there is effective discharge planning, those patients may not receive the treatment they need. This is particularly likely when there are no vacancies available in long-term care facilities. Specific cases of adverse treatment of patients, such as sending an eighty-one-year-old woman to a nursing home 183 miles away from her home have been identified (Baldwin 1985). Debates about the impact of the PPS on quality of care continue, with evidence from specific studies that support both the positions that there is an adverse effect and that there is no effect. A study of patients admitted with a diagnosis of hip fracture to a large community hospital, before and after the PPS was implemented, found a decline in the overall quality of care under the new system (Fitzgerald, Moore, and Dittus 1988). A different study of in-hospital deaths and readmissions during 1984 found no deterioration in the quality of care following the introduction of PPS, based on trends established before the new system (DesHarnais et al. 1987). A study of the effects of the PPS

88

in Rochester, New York concluded that the new system would not decrease quality of care if it were part of a community-wide planning effort for the delivery of health care services (Mushlin et al. 1988).

On balance, the new payment scheme does not seem, as a single factor, to lead to the deterioration in quality of care. If it is combined with decisions to discharge patients who cannot receive needed care outside of the hospital, however, it becomes one factor among several that can lower the quality of care received by the residents of a community.

The PPS can also have the unintended effect of limiting access to care. If the system, in an effort to induce efficiencies in all hospitals, forces some of the least efficient to close, it could have the effect of closing the only medical facility in some communities. This was a caution voiced after a study of the early experiences in New Jersey (Rosko 1984), and it is the primary concern of rural hospitals and their allies. Rural and inner-city hospitals have closed since the onset of the PPS, but the reasons for those closures are many and identifying the unique contribution of the PPS is difficult. Nonetheless, hospital closure has become a major political concern and steps have been taken to assist hospitals, both through the PPS and through other mechanisms that include direct grants and technical assistance. In the PPS, the designations of *rural referral center, sole community hospital,* and *disproportionate share* are intended to redress payment problems.

On balance, the PPS can be judged a success in reducing what would have been Medicare expenditures for inpatient hospital treatment. It can also be judged a success in containing overall Medicare expenditures. Thanks to this policy, Congress is able to use the Medicare program as a target for budget reductions each year when targets for deficit reduction must be met. The annual increase in Medicare hospital payments can be controlled by adjusting the PPS formula.

SUMMARY OF PPS

The prospective payment system will continue to be the method by which hospitals are reimbursed for services to Medicare patients, unless there is radical reform in health care finance. As long as the Prospective Payment Review Commission continues its work and the hospitals are represented in the health policy issue network, we should expect continued efforts to refine the system. The current effort, as of the winter of 1992, is to reclassify approximately one thousand rural hospitals as urban hospitals because their costs are close to those of urban hospitals. During 1992, the PPS will be modified to include payment for hospital capital expenses. Previously, those expenses continued to be reimbursed using a retrospective cost-based system. Once the change to prospective payment for capital expenses is completed, Congress can be expected to use that scheme as yet another tool to combat increasing expenditures and reduce budget deficits.

As the payment system continues to mature, hospital administrators and their staffs will find ways of working within the rules to increase their revenues. Some would argue that they have an unfair advantage over those who determine the rates, since resources for the bureaucracy administering the program are far fewer than those available to the industry (Sapolsky 1986). To the extent that payment objectives are met and hospital revenues are limited, a threat arises concerning the quality of care delivered. That is, if resources to hospitals are constrained severely beyond the abilities of hospital administrators to adjust through reduced costs, the level of services may suffer in order to compensate (Sapolsky 1986). There is a tenuous balance between quality and cost, and an emphasis on the latter may place the former at risk. Since payers have more representation in the health policy issue network than the recipients of care, and since the government itself is a major payer, the emphasis on cost containment will continue. The balance with quality is retained, to whatever extent it is, because of the political importance of two groups. First, certain groups of providers, most recently rural hospitals, have organized to voice a strong concern. Second, individual constituents can influence the judgment of legislators, such as the eighty-one-year-old woman forced to convalesce in a nursing home 183 miles from home. Specific cases such as this create powerful arguments for change because elected officials often respond most readily to real human concerns. Individuals affected by changes in public policy help illustrate the human impacts of those policies and call attention to deficiencies.

The emphasis on payment puts pressure on access. Public policymakers are beginning to recognize that if they want to pay for efficient care by setting a universal formula, they will have to subsidize some providers that simply cannot meet those standards of efficiency because of circumstances beyond their control (such as the size of the community where they practice). In sum, the use of the PPS has been a payment policy that has opened the policy debate to other concerns that had been disguised by the previous generous system of reimbursement.

Reform of Physician Reimbursement

The second largest component of health expenditures, after the share taken by hospitals, is the share for services provided directly by physicians. In the continuing effort to control expenditures in the Medicare program and for health care more generally, Congress has begun the process of changing the method used to pay physicians. In addition to controlling aggregate expenditures for physician services, the new methodology will serve the objective of changing the relative reimbursements for different subcategories of physicians, such as, paying more to family practice specialists and less to surgeons.

THE NEED FOR REFORM

Since the inception of Medicare in 1965, physicians have been paid according to calculations based on their historical charges. Physicians have been reimbursed "reasonable" charges for their services, based on the actual charge for the service, the physician's own customary charge for the service, and the "prevailing charge" for similar services in the local area (the nation is divided into 225 areas for the calculation). Allowable charges have been updated annually using an economic index devised for the Medicare program that accounts for changes in operating expenses and earning levels.

If the payers for care (such as Medicare and major third party insurers) could be confident that physicians were charging reasonable rates for their services, this historical system would be satisfactory. Such is not the case, however. Beginning in the early 1980s, the scheme of paying customary charges came under fire because physicians were "gaming" the system to maximize personal income. Some critics of the system were caustic: "The charges for medical services have escalated, with little or no restraint, to the point at which current fee levels in several medical and surgical specialties are simply indefensible and deserving of public censure" (Roe 1981, 41). Under the old system, physicians were able to continue to drive the customary fees to higher levels by simply increasing their charges.[1] Thus, by June 1980, the average fee paid by Blue Shield to the surgeon for services in coronary-bypass operations was between $3,500 and $4,200, which is an annual income of $350,000 from this operation (Roe 1981). The Medicare program pays, after a deductible paid by the individual, a percentage of the customary charges (usually 80 percent), so the total fees

1. Although they may not always be paid the full charges because in any given year, those could exceed the "customary" charges, the customary level in future years is affected by the *charge* in previous years, not the payments.

under that program are somewhat lower than those of private insurance. Nonetheless, the average fee paid to surgeons performing a coronary artery bypass with three grafts in 1985 was $3,714 (Cromwell et al. 1989).

While the PPS was being implemented by the Department of Health and Human Services, legislative attention turned to the problem of physician payment. The reason is evident when the increases in physician payments are reviewed. Aggregate Medicare spending on physicians' services increased by over 20 percent per year from 1979 through 1981, and by 19.8, 18.5, and 10.6 percent in 1982, 1983, and 1984, respectively. The increase in expenditures was a function of both the total services provided and the cost per service. The latter increased 13 percent for cardiovascular disease from 1975 to 1982, 13 percent for general surgery and ophthalmology, and 10 percent for dermatology, oncology, orthopedic surgery, and general practice (Etheredge and Juba 1984).

The first attack on physician payment was to freeze physicians' payments per service for fifteen months, as a provision of the Deficit Reduction Act of 1984. Congress also created a new classification of physicians—the "participating" physicians—who would accept Medicare reimbursement as payment in full (not billing patients for differences between payments and charges). The rules of the payment freeze were more liberal for participating physicians, and the freeze was lifted for them before it was for the remainder of physicians. Fees were again frozen in a provision of the Omnibus Budget Reconciliation Act of 1987, this time from January through March 1988.

When the PPS was adopted for hospitals in 1983, many analysts predicted that Congress would adopt a similar DRG-based reimbursement system to pay physicians. Designing a diagnosis-based system for physician services, however, would be a massive undertaking since the same diagnosis could indicate any of several actions. A better parameter would seem to be retaining a procedure-based system but finding a means other than historical charges for determining fair reimbursement rates for those procedures. Even at that, the task is rather daunting: in recent years Medicare received approximately 350 million claims a year from 500,000 physicians for 7,000 different procedures (Roper 1988).

THE EVOLUTION OF PAYMENT REFORM

In the Consolidated Omnibus Budget Reconciliation Act of 1985, Congress created the Physician Payment Review Commission (PPRC) and charged it with the responsibility of making recommendations concerning Medicare physicians' payments. The commission began in June 1986. The Commission was also to advise the secretary of DHHS in developing a relative-value scale (RVS) to pay for physicians' services. The Office of Research and Demonstrations, Health Care Financing Administration, contracted with a team of researchers at Harvard University (headed by Professor William Hsiao) to develop a resource-based relative-value scale (RBRVS) for use by Medicare. As in the case of hospital payment reform, Congress gave instructions concerning the general nature of the new system but left the specifics to an administrative agency, this time with the help of an independent commission.

While waiting for the final recommendations, Congress restricted payment for certain procedures already judged to be overpaid. In 1988, reductions were made in the payments for the following procedures: coronary artery bypass surgery, total hip replacement, cataract surgery, transurethral prostatectomy, suprapubic prostatectomy, knee arthroscopy, and knee arthroplasty (O'Sullivan 1988).

Developing a new payment system proved to be a long and difficult task. Professor Hsiao's work has been completed and there is now a methodology for determining fees for specific procedures. The building blocks of the methodology are the total work input of the physician, the costs of the physician's practice, and the cost of training (including opportunity costs). Physicians participated in the study to determine ratings of work efforts for specific procedures. Extensive personal interviews with physicians from a variety of specialties were conducted to determine the most important components of work efforts, and then ratings of actual work were gathered from a random sample of physicians using a telephone survey. A total of 1,977 physicians were interviewed for the study, creating a reliable estimate of the work effort involved in the complete array of services (Hsiao et al. 1988). An index can be used that incorporates the variables used in the Hsiao study to establish a value for each procedure reimbursed. Once that is done, a formula similar to that used in the PPS can be employed to determine the actual payment for each procedure.

The PPRC made its recommendation to adopt the Hsiao index, with modifications, in its third annual report to Congress in 1989. The modifications were to separate the cost of liability insurance from other costs of practice, to incorporate a measure of time in evaluation and management services, and to develop a uniform policy defining general fees for surgeons (Iglehart 1989b). Three years of work by the PPRC and by the Harvard team of researchers resulted in sufficient detail concerning implementation to provide impetus for Congress to act.

The decision-making locus in 1989 was clearly in Congress, and the response was to push forward to adopt the new system. The Omnibus Reconciliation Act of 1989 required that the resource-based relative-value scale (RBRVS) be in place by 1992 as the means by which Medicare would determine payment to physicians. As of this writing there are still details to be completed before the final implementation of the new system, and the political activity is intense.

Congress has been able to move forward with this complete restructuring of physician reimbursement for two reasons. The first is that the nature of the system creates winners and losers in the medical profession. For example, the income for physicians in rural areas will increase 15 percent, whereas their metropolitan counterparts would see a 14 percent decline (Stevens 1989b). Payments for internal medicine and family practice physicians will increase, while payments to general surgeons and radiologists will decrease (Stevens 1989b). The difference in impacts of the new payment system has made it difficult to mobilize significant opposition. Only when more sweeping effects are considered, such as restricting the total pool of funds for physician reimbursement, are organizations such as the American Medical Association able to mount effective efforts to resist the change. The AMA actually participated in the Hsiao study, whereas the American College of Surgeons, a group with a more narrowly defined membership that is affected adversely, has opposed it (Alston 1989). The positions of many medical professional societies have been to favor the concept of RBRVS while wanting to participate in how it is calculated for the procedures performed by their particular members. In a hearing before the Subcommittee on Health of the Committee on Ways and Means in the House of Representatives on 14 May 1988, the following associations testified in favor of RBRVS: The American Academy of Family Physicians, the American Society of Internal Medicine, and the American College of Physicians. Even the American College of Surgeons' testimony was careful to praise the general effort to change the Medicare payment system, while disagreeing strongly with the particulars of the PPRC recommendations (Austen 1988). The interests of physicians have been sufficiently splintered to minimize their influence in the issue network, opening an opportunity for those seeking reform, such as Representative Pete Stark (chair of the Ways and Means Subcommittee on Health), to prevail.

The second reason Congress has made progress in establishing a new scheme for reimbursing physicians is that the policy environment emphasizing budget deficit reduction increases the political appeal of any initiative that might contribute to that single policy objective. In that context, the evolution of physician payment policies in recent years is traced through amendments to the Deficit Reduction Act of 1984 and subsequent Omnibus Reconciliation Acts. These pieces of general legislation set the agenda for changing existing programs, including Medicare. Further, the efforts in physicians' payment reform have been defined either as budget-neutral or deficit-reduction mechanisms, making them germane to reconciliation legislation. The pressure to control costs has been intense and has created the opportunity for dramatic reform.

THE NEXT STEPS

The reform has occurred and will continue to occur, in incremental fashion, in the following steps: The first step was to freeze physicians' payments, creating pressure to find a mutually agreed-upon (between physicians and Congress) means of establishing fair payments. The second step was to create incentives for physicians to accept Medicare payments as payment in full for Medicare patients. The third step was to support activities to change the reimbursement system. The fourth step was to limit payments of certain procedures, creating the precedent to reduce some payments. Finally, Congress moved to a wholesale change of the reimbursement system, but even that change will initially be budget neutral and has undergone modification to reduce the losses to some groups of medical professionals.

Some important issues continue to plague Congress as the implementation date for the new system draws nearer. Then Director of the Health Care Financing Administration (HCFA) William Roper raised some concerns in 1988 that the new system might limit payment per procedure but continued growth in the volume and intensity of services would inspire continued rapid growth in aggregate physicians' payments (Roper 1988). The PPRC and others have recommended that the new system include expenditure targets to limit the total volume of payments (Alston 1989). If expenditure targets are included, they will be enforced by reducing the payment rates following any year in which targets are exceeded.

Other problems also remain. The complete list of rates for all 7,400 procedures reimbursed by Medicare is not yet available. However, 2,700 procedures have been priced, and they represent 95 percent of all Medicare spending. The measurement of geographic variations also needs to be refined (PPRC is working on this); and variations in labor costs, complexity, and technological advances still need to be calculated and built into the payment formula, which will be a conversion factor to convert efforts established by RBRVS into real dollars in payment for services (Wiener 1991b). During the next year or two we will see the preimplementation politics take place as professional groups attempt to maximize their returns from the new system. After that, issues of quality and access similar to those raised following PPS will be raised concerning physician care.

SUMMARY OF PHYSICIAN'S PAYMENT POLICIES

Until the late 1980s, physicians were not a notable target for budget-cutting efforts, since health care expenditures for their services were so much lower than those being paid to hospitals. With the advent of the PPS, however, members of Congress and others in the issue network concerned about continued increases in health expenditures looked to physicians' fees as the next place to restrain the continual growth. Physicians have long had a powerful presence in the health policy issue network, through the lobbying efforts of the AMA. How then can physician expenditures be controlled with legislative initiatives that could be opposed by the AMA?

Physicians were included in the development of a new payment system, giving them a stake in the success of that effort. Many groups of physicians, including those practicing in rural areas and primary care physicians, will gain income as a result of a new payment scheme. Opposition remains among physicians, with practitioners of certain specialties such as surgery objecting to the reductions in income they expect to result from the new system. Greater opposition has mobilized physicians to fight particular elements of the new system, especially suggestions that the formula be used as a means of limiting all Medicare expenditures for physicians' care to levels well below those that would otherwise occur. Physicians have supported the new system as a rational means of determining payment for services rendered; their support was not offered in order to use this system as a tool to reduce deficit spending.

Health policy, as related to reimbursement, has become intertwined with budget policy since 1983. After careful development of a new physicians' payment system, including participation of policy analysts such as William Hsiao, the particulars of implementation are being clouded by the interest of others in the network, particularly the executive branch, to use this health policy tool to accomplish budget objectives. The same characteristic of the policy environment that helped create the opportunity to change physicians' payment may delay its implementation.

Other Cost-Containment Efforts

Prospective-payment and relative-value scales have been the buzzwords of cost containment in recent years, but those two major efforts have not been the only policies aimed at cost control. For example, in the early years of PPS, four states (New York, New Jersey, Massachusetts, and Maryland) were given waivers from the federal program because they had adopted cost-containment programs of their own, which included all sources of payment for hospital care. Those states were just as successful as PPS in restraining growth in Medicare costs, at the same time enabling more effective control of Medicaid expenditures. In addition, commercial insurers in those states were more competitive with Blue Cross (Zuckerman and Holahan 1988).

Private insurers and self-insured corporations are also actively trying to control health care expenditures. Several strategies have been used by private groups: negotiations with hospitals and doctors, rewarding employees who do not spend all of the expected funds, using managed care to increase efficiencies, and adopting wellness and other programs to keep employees healthy (Gray 1989). In addition to the four PPS waiver states described earlier, other state governments have been adopting cost control mechanisms. A number of states have incorporated utilization review (a check on the necessity of hospital admissions) and managed care into their Medicaid programs. Other efforts include the following: direct purchase of vaccines from the Centers for Disease Control; competitive bidding for laboratory services, oxygen services, wheelchairs, and home care; prospective pricing for Medicaid services; and selective contracting for Medicaid services (*HealthWeek* Staff, 1990b).

Efforts to contain health care costs can be expected to continue, and they are as various as the payers for health care services. In view of continuous increases in aggregate expenditures, those efforts seem to do little more than chip away at the edges of this growing monolith.

Conclusions

Cost containment remains a high priority of public policy related to health care delivery. Fiscal pressures on public budgets, be they the federal government and the Medicare program or the states and the Medicaid program, are intensifying annually. Major changes in hospital payment, and, in the near future, physician payment, will have some effect on expenditures, but they have not been able to stem the tide. What is to be done?

There are three major options. The first is to simply accept the high costs of medical care as expenses that can be absorbed by the citizens of the United States. This choice would avoid decisions to restrict the incomes of medical care providers and/or limit the services available to any citizens. Justification for this nonaction would be based on the fact that there are still other major categories of "waste" in the use of the nation's domestic product, such as the consumption of cigarettes and alcohol, which actually help drive the increases in health expenditures.

A second option is to continue to chip away at the causes of health expenditure increases, with a combination of public and private initiatives. Each of these initiatives seems to have at least some limited effect. Since they generally focus on only one set of providers and/or actions at a time, however, it is far too easy to simply shift expenditures to another segment of the health care delivery system. If some payers for care are completely successful in controlling all the expenses for the persons they finance, expenditures can be shifted to other payers.

A third option would be to change radically the system for insuring health care and/or to ration health care services. A radical change in health insurance would entail creating a single national plan, so that a single payer could negotiate with health care providers and thereby achieve cost savings. The ability to pass costs on to other payers would be eliminated. Further, if the insurance plan paid for all services, the ability to shift expenses to other providers or settings would also be eliminated. Another approach to radical change would be to ration health care. The experiment under way in the state of Oregon rations health care, after a systematic ranking of all possible health care services by priority according to their greatest benefits to the state's citizens. Another approach to rationing would be to limit the development and application of new technologies that are costly but of questionable marginal benefit (Callahan 1990).

Cost-containment policies have been developed only after experimentation, evaluation, and debate. The experimentation has occurred at state and local levels, where such ideas as prospective payment have been tried. Those experiments are evaluated by policy analysts before the specifics of national legislation are formulated. Even after an idea has been tried and proved to be successful, a great deal of political work remains before a national policy is adopted. Members of the health policy issue network will want to have input, protecting their own best interests. A key driving force behind cost-containment policies in the 1990s is the widespread admission that the current growth in total health care expenditures is not acceptable. Many in Congress and elsewhere would argue that the nation now faces a crisis in health care expenditures. If that argument is accepted, decision makers may not wait for careful elaboration, experimentation, and evaluation of new ideas to contain costs. Instead, radical changes in payment policies may be adopted in the hopes that the cost curve can be contained.

Before adopting any further steps to control health expenditures, trade-offs with other objectives should be considered. For every effort to control costs there are risks to the objectives of quality and access. Unless costs are controlled, however, providing universal access will be difficult if not impossible, and the best quality of care the system can provide may be realized only by the few who can afford the charges.

The complex nature of health care delivery can be both a blessing and a curse to efforts to contain cost increases. Increased and intense competition among providers may lead to more efficient delivery of care. Purchasers of health care services, either individuals or groups, may be able to shop around to secure the greatest return for their health care dollar. For example, if an HMO provides high quality medical care for less than is charged by private practice physicians, consumers can enroll in HMOs. If outpatient surgery is more cost effective than being admitted as a patient to a hospital, benefits in insurance programs can encourage the former. The wide variety of possible services, though, can be a hindrance to cost-containment efforts. If public policies are designed to control costs in a particular modality of delivering medical care, providers can simply shift their work efforts to a different modality that still pays them more.

For those providers unable to shift their work to more profitable delivery modalities, and for communities unable to attract the most efficient modes of delivering care, uniform pricing rules that control costs by restraining charges for certain services may eliminate access to health care. If providers can no longer provide services and earn a reasonable living, they are likely to shift to locations and practices that will generate greater income. Policies designed to take advantage of innovations in health care delivery, such as HMOs and free-standing surgical centers, may work to the disadvantage of small rural communities unable to attract those types of providers. In short, we continue to walk the fine line, balancing the goals of cost containment, quality, and access.

5

· · ·

Issues in Access
to Health Care

As we move toward the next century, public concern is mounting about problems American citizens experience in attempting to access the health care system. To the surprise of some who in the late 1980s viewed access as a minor concern when compared to cost containment, as of September 1992 more than twenty-five different bills intended to increase the number of Americans with health insurance coverage were introduced in the 102d Congress. A large number of persons without any form of health insurance and the increasing public awareness of that problem, combined with a fear that "this could happen to me," are creating a policy environment conducive to discussions of government policies to expand access.

Access problems can be geographic as well as financial. Beginning in the second half of the 1980s, members of Congress expressed strong interest in addressing problems of providing adequate and high-quality medical care in rural areas. Coalitions were formed in both the House and the Senate to advocate legislation favorable to rural health, and there are stronger advocates among the interest groups in the health policy issue network. The changes in the network helped change the policy environment, creating opportunities for policies that work in rural areas.

The U.S. Congress and state legislatures have been considering and enacting policies designed to redress the problems documented in this chapter. The efforts have been the typical incremental responses to crises, however, not designed to eradicate entire problems. The problems continue and for some groups of citizens they are worsening. Therefore, despite strong pressures to control health care expenditures, we should expect more policies designed to expand access to health care.

The Problems of the Uninsured

As a society we ought to be concerned that in 1987, 10 percent of impaired children, those who need special medical attention, were uninsured and that Medicaid covered only 60 percent of poor disabled children (Davis 1987). Regardless of our views about the merits of providing financial assistance to the poor, few of us want to ignore the health needs of the nation's youth. Since 1987 the situation has improved for children, thanks to federal initiatives in the budget reconciliation acts of recent years. Nevertheless, millions of Americans, including children, lack any form of health insurance (including Medicare and Medicaid). For those persons, access to health care services is not assured, and as a result many suffer from maladies that may have been prevented or at least eased considerably. There have been some policy initiatives in recent years to address this problem, including national policies to expand Medicaid eligibility for children and various state policies to provide health insurance benefits to those previously uninsured.

THE NUMBER AND CHARACTERISTICS OF THE UNINSURED

Estimates of the total number of Americans without any form of public or private insurance vary, between thirty-three million and thirty-eight million. The variation is a function of how the uninsured are counted (using particular questions in surveys of Americans), but all surveys are in agreement that the number has increased in recent years, and it remains high (Swartz 1990). Numbers will be reported here from the three most widely used national sources: the 1987 National Medical Expenditures Survey (NMES), the 1989 National Health Interview Survey (NHIS), and the Current Population Survey (CPS) from March of various years. The first survey was conducted by the Agency for Health Care Policy and Research, U. S. Department of Health and Human Services (DHHS); the second by the National Center for Health Statistics, DHHS; and the last by the U.S. Bureau of the Census. Levels of uninsurance from Michigan, Ohio, and Nebraska will also be reported. Table 5.1 reports the results from those surveys and from reports of uninsurance rates in separate states.

If the number of uninsured people indicates a temporary problem, perhaps related to a downturn in the nation's economy, policy interventions could be minimal. The problem is far more serious, however. Although rates of uninsur-

Table 5.1 Rates of Uninsurance

Source of Data	National Rate* (%)	Number	State Rate* (%)
NMES 1987	15.5	36.8 million	
CPS 1990	16.1	34.4 million	
NHIS 1989	15.7	33.9 million	
Michigan 1987		860,000	10.8
Ohio 1985		1.36 million	14.4
Nebraska 1990		142,000	11.4

*Rates are a percent of the number of persons under the age of 65; less than 2 percent of those over 65 are not insured because of ineligibility for Social Security benefits.

Sources: Short et al. 1988; Foley 1991; Ries 1991; GAO 1990 and 1988; Blankenau, Holder, and Mueller 1991.

ance in 1987 were lower than those of the recession years of the mid-1980s, they remained quite high; in 1985 the national rate was 18 percent, compared with 17 percent in 1987; whereas the comparable figures in Michigan were 12 and 11 percent (GAO 1990, 6). Analysis of the results of survey research in Nebraska indicates that what might be termed the *base line* rate of uninsurance, the rate we should expect when the economy is at full strength, has increased considerably since the early 1980s. Even though 1990 was the best year of the previous eleven in per capita income and employment, the rate of uninsurance was the highest for those years (Blankenau, Holder, and Mueller 1991). The contrast between the improving situation in unemployment and the worsening situation in uninsurance is dramatic (see figure 5.1 and table 5.2). As evident in the CPS data, the same leveling and slightly worsening situation is true nationally although not as dramatic in impact.

Why is the rate of uninsurance high and staying there? That question can be answered by examining the characteristics of the uninsured populations, and those variables that are statistically related to the rate of uninsurance. A high percentage of the uninsured reside in households in which at least one adult works at least part-time (see table 5.3).

Employees in small firms are the least likely to be insured, and those employed in seasonal jobs, agriculture, construction, and sales, were less likely to be insured than persons in other occupations (Short, Monheit, and Beauregard 1988). Being employed provides no guarantee of being insured. Although persons with incomes below poverty are the most likely to be uninsured (37 percent of that group in 1987), those between poverty and twice poverty level incomes are also at a high rate of uninsurance (29 percent in 1987) (GAO 1989). The same

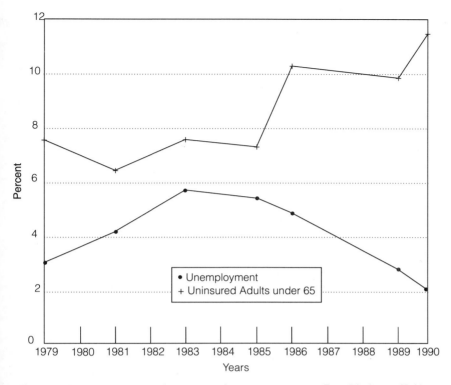

Figure 5.1. Unemployment and uninsurance, various years, 1979–1990. From Blankenau, Holder, and Mueller 1991.

pattern holds in Michigan, where the likelihood of being uninsured is 26 percent under poverty and 20 percent between poverty and twice that income level. In Nebraska, similar numbers have been reported in 1990: 31.9 percent of households with incomes below $5,000 include uninsured members, 27.9 percent with incomes between $5,000 and $9,999, and 19.4 percent with incomes between $10,000 and $14,999 (Blankenau, Holder, and Mueller 1991). Many of the jobs created since the recession of the mid-1980s have been in small businesses and in the service sector of the economy; they have not typically been jobs that included health insurance benefits as part of their compensation packages. In short, there seems to be little if any cause for optimism—this problem is here to stay until resolved by comprehensive policy solutions.

The magnitude of the problem of access for the uninsured is more apparent when more specific numbers are examined. For example, in 1987, approximately 17 percent of women of childbearing age had no health insurance

Table 5.2 Uninsurance Rates among Respondents under Age 65 and Margin of Error for Selected Years, 1979–1990

Year	Uninsurance Rate (%)	Margin of Error (%)
1979	7.6	+/– 1.3
1981	6.6	+/– 1.3
1983	7.6	+/– 1.3
1985	7.5	+/– 1.3
1986	10.2	+/– 1.5
1989	9.9	+/– 1.5
1990	11.4	+/– 1.5

Source: Blankenau, Holder, and Mueller 1991.

Table 5.3 Employment Characteristics of Households with Uninsured Members

Year	Households with Employed Adult (%)	Households with Full-Time Employed Adult (%)
1987	70	46.3
1989	89	54

Sources: Short, Monheit, and Beauregard 1988; Foley 1991.

(Barber-Madden and Kotch 1990). The unfortunate implication is that those women may lack access to prenatal care and/or fertility services. For the over 30 million Americans without health insurance, all medical expenses are their own responsibility. They must pay medical debts as best they can, as was the case for a self-employed Washington, D.C., construction worker who fell from scaffolding and incurred a hospital emergency room bill for hundreds of dollars (Rich 1990). The uninsured are, for the most part, the nation's working poor.

ACCESS PROBLEMS AMONG THE UNINSURED

Being without health insurance often means being without medical care, either by force or by choice. One woman interviewed by reporter Spencer Rich reported not getting periodic check-ups because she could not afford them; another said she did not see the doctor unless the problem was very serious (Rich 1990). In a survey in 1986, the Robert Wood Johnson Foundation found that 31 percent of the uninsured lacked a regular source of care compared with 16 percent of the insured (Robert Wood Johnson Foundation 1987). Individual stories of poor health outcomes for financial reasons are being reported. One of the most dramatic is the tale of a man who died of a malignant melanoma after delaying care because he could not afford it. Another person reported to *Consumer Affairs* that a hospital would not admit his wife for a cancer operation because he could not prepay $7,000 (Karpatkin 1991). Such tragedies are reported to Congress in public hearings and to the general public as special news stories. Because of these specific cases that illustrate the general problem, the policy environment is changing to emphasize access problems.

The plight of those without insurance during the 1980s became particularly acute when public programs that had served as their safety net were cut. For example, over 250 community health centers closed after funding cuts in 1982, and the Women, Infants, and Children nutrition programs in 1985 had funds sufficient to meet only one third of the estimated need (Mundinger 1985).

Evidence has been reported that links lack of insurance coverage with lower percentages of Pap smears and breast examinations among women (Braveman et al. 1988). A 1986 survey of maternal and child health agencies in the fifty states and the District of Columbia revealed the following: in fifteen states hospitals denied admission to women about to deliver; in thirteen states hospitals denied admission to women not in "active" labor; and six state agencies were aware of patient dumping (transfers from one hospital to another) (Rosenbaum, Hughes, and Johnson 1988). Although there have been actions both by the federal government through Medicare and by states through regulatory policies to prevent hospitals' refusals to treat patients in emergencies (Hudson 1988), the financial incentives to avoid treating those unable to pay are obvious, and evidence shows providers will avoid those patients if possible. A U.S. General Accounting Office study in eight states found that 63 percent of the women surveyed, mostly uninsured or receiving Medicaid, were not obtaining sufficient prenatal care (Oberg 1990).

The evidence that the uninsured receive quantitatively less care than the insured is compelling, both in samples of the nation's general population (Freeman et al. 1990) and in samples of particular populations, such as the nation's adult blacks (Neighbors and Jackson 1987). From the evidence just presented, we know that the uninsured receive less care and at times are denied access to particular health care providers. Do these problems in access have any particular adverse consequences to the ultimate outcome, the health of the individual (including birth outcomes)? The examples presented earlier are concrete illustrations that they do.

Others have reached the same conclusion after examining evidence concerning groups of the uninsured. A study of hospital discharge data in the San Francisco area covering over two years demonstrated that lack of insurance was "associated significantly with adverse hospital outcomes" and that the effects were worse among Latinos (Braveman et al. 1989). This finding indicates a compound cultural and economic barrier to care. Another California study followed health access patterns and outcomes for a population that was removed from the Medi-Cal program and left uninsured. After one year, 68 percent reported an episode when they felt they needed care but did not get it, and 78 percent of them listed cost as the reason. Most dramatically, after examining seven deaths, "lack of access to care played a part in at least four of the deaths in the medically indigent group" (Lurie et al. 1986).

The individual cases of ill health and even death are calling public attention to the problem of uninsurance and the personal problems that result. Studies with larger samples of the uninsured are being reported that increase our knowledge of the scope of the problem. The adverse consequences of uninsurance create a policy environment that facilitates action. Policy analysts in the issue network are examining the reasons for persons not having insurance, and suggestions for policy follow from those explanations. The next step is policy action.

POLICIES TO PROVIDE ACCESS FOR THE UNINSURED

The most radical policy suggestions to resolve this problem are those calling for a single system of national health insurance, and they will be discussed in chapter 7. There are other policies to consider nationally that would address the needs of various groups of persons among the uninsured, and they will be discussed briefly in the following paragraphs. Much of the current public policy action, though, is taking place within various states, so those policies will receive more extensive discussion in this chapter. Finally, there may be approaches to expanding the reach of health insurance through private initiatives, and they too will be described.

Since 1984, policies have been enacted by Congress which expand Medicaid eligibility requirements to allow for more participation of children in the program. In 1984, the first steps were to mandate coverage of pregnant women and children in two-parent families who met income eligibility requirements and to mandate coverage for all children five years old or younger who meet financial eligibility requirements. When the federal government mandates Medicaid eligibility or benefits, it is in effect telling the states that they must expand their programs accordingly to continue receiving federal matching dollars. Thus,

Congress can use this device as a means of sharing the cost of increasing access with the states. The states, on the other hand, have no choice but to add the new categories of individuals to the Medicaid rolls, increasing their costs without controlling the decision. In 1986, states were given the option of covering pregnant women and children up to five years of age in families with incomes below 100 percent of federal poverty, regardless of their participation in the Aid to Dependent Children (ADC) program; in 1988 that option was increased to 185 percent of federal poverty income. In 1988, as part of the Medicare Catastrophic Act that remains in effect, Congress mandated coverage for pregnant women and infants in families with incomes below 100 percent of federal poverty guidelines, and in 1989, that was expanded to 133 percent of poverty and children to the age of six years. Finally, in 1988, Congress required that Medicaid coverage be continued for six months for families leaving the ADC program and allowed states the option of adding six months to that extension.

A key element in these incremental expansions of federal involvement in Medicaid as a program for the poor has been the erosion of the traditional eligibility linkage between Medicaid and AFDC. Requiring participation in the latter program has in the past severely restricted the number of poor persons participating in Medicaid (in 1989 less than 50 percent of the nation's poor were eligible for Medicaid benefits). One barrier created by linking the programs is a requirement that income be far less than federal poverty guidelines, since states set eligibility for AFDC at very low income levels. In Alabama, for example, the income requirement is $118 a month or less for a family of three, or 13 percent of poverty (Pepper Commission 1990). The plight of the poor trying to obtain Medicaid benefits has worsened in recent years, with the median state AFDC level dropping 30 percent in real dollars between 1970 and 1988 (Pepper Commission 1990). In addition to income eligibility restrictions, Medicaid requirements have limited benefits to families with only one adult in the household. The new provisions passed by Congress since 1984 have provided precedent to break these longtime linkages to the AFDC program, at least for pregnant women and children (Pear 1988).

Changes in Medicaid rules in recent years signal an improvement in access to care, but they are consistent with the program's limited objectives: "Medicaid was never designed to serve everyone who is poor, nor to meet all the health care needs of those eligible" (Tallon 1990, 6). By allowing children to be covered, even if the family is not eligible for AFDC benefits, Medicaid will provide an opportunity for access for an entire segment of the poor population. Opportunity, however, does not necessarily guarantee actual access, and certainly not access to high-quality care. In the nation's urban areas, overburdened private physicians create Medicaid "mills" to process a large number of patients in a short time. By doing so, the physician is assured of an adequate income even though the payment per person served is low. The poor, though, do not receive adequate care under these conditions. All complaints are treated the same, and diagnostic measures often include only taking the patient's temperature and hearing the general complaint (Specter 1991).

A study of responses to a national survey completed in 1988 found that children eligible for Medicaid received more services than other poor children, but that they received those services in community clinics, not private physicians' offices. Access through the Medicaid program is to a different source of medical care than that available to privately insured children (St. Peter, Newacheck, and Halfon 1992). Moreover, expanding Medicaid eligibility is no guarantee of increased use of medical services. A study of clients eligible for Medicaid completed in Tennessee after changes in Medicaid eligibility in 1985 found no changes in birth weight, neonatal mortality, or the use of early prenatal care, (Piper, Ray, and Griffin 1990).

The Medicaid program is a vehicle for incremental change but not for assuring access to medical care for the nation's uninsured. Among the uninsured are millions of Americans who would not be categorically eligible for services, adults with no dependent children. Additionally, unless the linkage to AFDC is broken for all clients, states are unlikely to increase income limits to the current poverty level, much less above that amount as required to encompass most of the uninsured population. The barrier to using Medicaid is straightforward: providing Medicaid benefits to all the uninsured with incomes below 200 percent of federal poverty guidelines could double federal and state expenditures for this program. Even if the expansion of Medicaid eligibility were limited to all of the uninsured with incomes below 75 percent of poverty, government expenditures for the program could increase by as much as 45 percent ($11.5 billion in 1991 dollars) (Holahan and Zedlewski 1991). In lieu of this fiscal reality, incremental changes in the program are the only likely policy choice.

Responding incrementally to a serious problem is the typical legislative preference, and such has been the case with the issue of uninsurance in recent years. Actions have been taken on behalf of poor women and children, yet the problem of over thirty-three million Americans with no health insurance remains. What will the national government do next to address the problem? The U.S. Bipartisan Commission on Comprehensive Health Care, better known as the Pepper Commission, released its recommendations in September 1990, and they constitute at least one starting point for debate in the halls of Congress and elsewhere. Demonstrating how difficult action in this area will prove to be in Congress, the commission, composed of members of Congress in influential committee positions and three private experts, supported the recommendations on access to care by the narrow margin of 8 to 7.

Those voting against the final recommendations nevertheless recognized the seriousness of the problem and the need for action. The commission's recommendations were to require that health insurance coverage be offered by employers of more than fifty persons and to provide incentives to employers of less than fifty persons to provide health insurance, requiring them to do so after a reasonable time to adjust to this expense. The commission also recommended that the federal government replace and expand Medicaid to cover all groups not covered through employment-based insurance (Pepper Commission 1990, 7). Members of Congress, including Senator John D. (Jay) Rockefeller, who chaired the commission, have proposed specific legislation implementing the commission's recommendations.

Congress has demonstrated the desire and political will to address the needs of a small number of the uninsured perceived to be the most vulnerable—pregnant women and children—but has not developed a consensus on more dramatic steps to move beyond incremental adjustments to existing programs. Participants in the issue network, as shown in the votes of the Pepper Commission, cannot agree on a single approach to resolve the problem. In fact, some debate continues about just how serious the problem is, with DHHS Secretary Sullivan saying that we should be focusing on the access needs of a subset of the uninsured, because access is not a problem for all thirty-one to thirty-seven million of the uninsured (Wiener 1991a). With the national government confronting a budget crisis, dramatic and costly initiatives are not likely to be enacted. Given the changes in the policy environment, however, such measures may be introduced now in order to refine them and be ready for further consideration later. During the 102d Congress, several such proposals were introduced, including Health Act USA by Senator Kerrey of Nebraska and the Comprehensive Care for All Americans Act by Representative Oakar of Ohio. The issue network is primed to debate the provisions of such programs, even before the policymakers are ready to move to adopt them.

Incremental adjustments have already been made, and more are likely to follow. Long-term precedents linking health care benefits to welfare programs have been broken and could be shattered with further action to broaden Medicaid benefits to different income groups and to families with both adults still in the household. Additional incremental change could begin to provide incentives to employers to offer health insurance as a precursor to eventually requiring such coverage. Several states are experimenting with programs, funded by the Robert Wood Johnson Foundation, to increase the availability of insurance through small employers. As of mid-1992, these programs had enrolled less than 10 percent of the uninsured populations in their states, and increases in the costs of insurance premiums continued to act as barriers to providing insurance (Helms, Gauthier, and Campion 1992).

Most of the incremental actions of recent years, and certainly those that are to come in the near future, originate in state governments. State government officials recognize the simple truth of American federalism: they are the principal line of attack against social problems such as access to care for the uninsured—they "are on the firing line" (statement of National Governors' Association chairman Governor Gardner of Washington, quoted in Lemov 1990). Similar to federal efforts, various states have taken incremental actions designed to meet the needs of the most vulnerable of the uninsured.

One action, taken by twenty-four states so far, is to create a special program, a "risk pool," to help persons acquire private insurance who are otherwise unable to do so because of the medical risks they pose to insurance companies. Most of these programs are financed by a combination of individual premiums and taxes on insurance carriers. These programs provide a mechanism for small employers to offer insurance to all employees except those with high medical risks, knowing there is a state-supported option for the latter individuals and families. As of the end of 1988, there were 32,159 participants in these programs—clearly not a large percentage of the uninsured but nevertheless an important group because of their vulnerability to high medical expenditures.

Other state-initiated programs have addressed additional vulnerable populations. New Jersey recently began a program to assure access to care for all pregnant women: the Maternity Outreach and Managed Services Program. It is targeted to all women whose household income is less than 250 percent of federal poverty guidelines. The program combines with an existing program, Healthstart, which provides free prenatal care and preventive services for children under age two for families eligible for Medicaid (Sylvester 1990). The new program is financed with revenue from a special trust fund that also reimburses hospitals for uncompensated care. Florida is beginning a program that links health insurance to schools, Healthy Kids Corporation. It includes immunizations and screening, physician office visits, hospitalization, emergency services, maternity care, and other services for reduced fees ($11.46 per month for screening and immunizations, $52.82 per month for the other services) (Wilson 1991). Washington is developing a special program for the working poor that uses health maintenance organizations (HMOs) and preferred provider organizations (PPOs) to provide care within counties in the state. As of 1990, the Basic Health Plan had enrolled 8,200 members in five counties (O'Connor 1990). Maine has established a program, MaineCare, to offer HMO-based coverage at moderate prices to businesses with fifteen or fewer employees. The state will subsidize premiums on a sliding scale based on the ability of the employer to contribute (Lemov 1990). Minnesota has created a program called Children's Health Plan, which is designed to provide benefits to children up to age nine who live in families with incomes below 185 percent of poverty but who do not qualify for Medicaid, and Colorado and New York have recently enacted similar legislation (Lemov 1990).

Three states (Massachusetts, Hawaii, and Oregon) have been experimenting with much more comprehensive programs designed to provide universal access to care within their jurisdictions. The most widely known of these efforts is the Massachusetts plan, signed into law in 1988 and designed to become fully operational in 1992. It is a combination of mandating employment-based insurance and providing comprehensive benefits through the state to those not able to secure insurance through an employer (Colburn 1988). That program began with great fanfare and promise during the presidential election year of 1988 but has since faltered because of Massachusetts's declining economy, which has severely restricted revenues for the state government. In fact, current predictions are that the program will never be fully implemented (Mullen 1991).

A similar program in Hawaii has been successful, but its success is linked in part to a waiver of a federal law exempting employers from regulations on self-insurance policies (those that do not use insurance companies and instead finance the policies themselves). This waiver of the provisions of the Employee Retirement Insurance Security Act was granted by Congress as a single-state exemption when the legislation was enacted. In Hawaii, all employers must offer health insurance, and the policies must include at least a basic set of benefits. In addition, the state has expanded its Medicaid program to close the remaining gap after the mandates, resulting in a drop of uninsurance from 17 percent of its nonelderly population in the 1970s to 5 percent in 1989 (Lemov 1990). Finally, a new program is being shaped to reach that last 5 percent of uninsured persons.

Oregon has begun a new program that would provide universal coverage but not for all health care services. In order to make a universal program affordable, the benefits would be restricted to those services the state could afford. A budget would be set, then applied to a listing of health services ordered according to their benefits. A line would be drawn on that list to indicate those services that would be covered under the new program (Mayer and Kimball 1991). That program is still in the formulation stage and will require a special waiver from the federal government in order to use Medicaid funds. In 1992 the Bush administration denied the waiver.

Although exciting initiatives are being undertaken by state governments, only a handful offer hope for anything approximating universal coverage. Most of the policies are incremental steps to provide coverage to narrowly defined population groups. Once again, the common characteristics of the policy system are evident in the actions being taken. The likelihood of comprehensive action being taken by the states has to be considered bleak, given the realities of the fiscal crunch that is once again infecting many of the states. Even incremental changes in Medicaid, as represented by the recent federal mandates, are threatened by fiscal realities (Kimball 1991).

Another incremental response to the problems of the uninsured is exhibited by actions in the private sector to expand health insurance coverage. There are a few basic models that employers and others should follow to make health insurance more affordable for small groups presently having difficulty securing benefits. Multiple-employer trusts could be formed for the purpose of securing group benefits (Bjovberg 1986). Another option would be to form groups not associated with the workplace, such as farmers organizations and professional associations. These organizations currently make some health insurance coverage, particularly catastrophic coverage, available to members.

The principle activity of private insurers and employers in expanding health care benefits has been to contribute to resolving the problem of affordability. Private firms are increasingly adopting schemes to contain costs, most particularly bargaining on behalf of their insurees with medical professionals for reduced charges, which in turn allows for more affordable insurance premiums. The challenge to public policymakers is to help employers find affordable health care coverage, even if that means a difference in state-mandated benefits or changes in state and federal tax laws. If incremental approaches continue to be the favored responses to the problems of the uninsured, all three players—state governments, national government, and private employers—will have to continue their separate and coordinated efforts to help those in need of access to the system.

Access Problems for the Elderly

Since the Medicare program began in 1965, the health care problems of the elderly have been the subject of public policy, with two concerns dominating annual debates about Medicare policy: the need to restrain spending in order to keep the program viable, and the desire to make the program truly comprehensive by adding services not currently covered. Both concerns begin with the assumption that the elderly need public insurance in order to finance health care.

THE NEEDS OF THE ELDERLY

Life expectancy in the United States is at an all-time high, and as a result the percent and number of elderly citizens increases annually. In 1988, there were 28.5 million Americans over age sixty-four (12 percent of the total population), a figure projected to grow to 52.3 million (17 percent) by the year 2020 (Brody 1988). Within this broadly defined group of the elderly, the subgroup of the very oldest (those eight-five years old and older) is increasing at least as rapidly, projected to grow from 2.5 million persons in 1980 to 24 million by the year 2040 (Schneider 1989).

Although the percentage of the elderly with incomes below federal poverty guidelines is less than that among the nonelderly, the percentage with incomes between 100 percent and 200 percent of the poverty guideline is higher (Holden and Smeeding 1990). These elderly citizens are at economic risk of incurring large expenses for which they are not insured. Their risk is greater than that of either the very poor or the wealthy, and they are susceptible particularly to high costs related to long-term care. Approximately 60 percent of the elderly are in this income group (Holden and Smeeding 1990).

Benefits available through the Medicare program assist the elderly in obtaining health care by removing many of the financial barriers, but not all forms of care are included as Medicare benefits. For example, Medicare does not pay for services designed to prevent the onset of serious medical problems: "The lack of reimbursement for preventative services in Medicare is shortsighted and costly. It would seem, to use an analogy, that we would rather pay to replace the engine, than to occasionally check the oil" (Pawlson 1988). Medicare does not include reimbursement for prescription medication or for long-term care not rendered as posthospitalization rehabilitation.

In an effort to close the gap between what is reimbursed by Medicare and what is actually charged for health care services rendered, many of the nation's elderly purchase supplemental insurance from private carriers. In 1986, 71 percent of the elderly did so, and another 9 percent were covered for those expenses by Medicaid. That left 20 percent with no insurance against medical expenses not covered by Medicare. As a result, the elderly spent over 11 percent of their incomes for health care in 1989, an increase from 9 percent in 1972 (Levit and Cowan 1991). Among poor elderly (those with incomes at or below federal poverty level) without Medicaid coverage, two-thirds spend more than 15 percent of their incomes and on average spend 25 percent on medical services. Among the elderly with incomes slightly higher than poverty level, one third have incomes below poverty after paying medical expenses (Rowland and Lyons 1987). A privately funded study using data from the Consumer Expenditure Survey conducted by the U.S. Bureau of the Census revealed the following facts about spending for medical care by the elderly in 1991:

• The elderly spent nearly twice as much for health care as they did in 1961, $3,305 versus $1,589 (in inflation-adjusted dollars) per elderly family

• Health expenditures consume 17.1 percent of after-tax income for the average elderly family, compared to 10.6 percent in 1961.

• Spending for Medicare premiums increased 50 percent in real dollars from 1972 to 1991 (Families USA Foundation 1992).

For the 8.5 million elderly Americans living alone, 20 percent rely only on Medicare for health expense reimbursement. Among this group, medical expenses force 680,000 persons into poverty annually (Kasper 1988).

MEDICARE AND THE GAPS

In searching for incremental solutions to the access problems facing the elderly, the natural starting place is the Medicare program. We should recognize that the current program is limited, both in hospitalization benefits and in reimbursement for services rendered outside of the hospital. In Part A of the program all hospital services are covered, after payment of a single annual deductible of $592 (in 1990). Hospitals are reimbursed according to the amounts determined through the prospective payment system (PPS), and the elderly are not liable for any remaining charges. Part A of the program covers up to 150 days of skilled nursing facility care, provided the facility is certified by Medicare and that the patient is eligible for services (being recently discharged from a hospital). The elderly are liable for a copayment of 20 percent for nursing facility stays. Limited coverage for home health care visits is included in Part A for those who are qualified as a result of their medical conditions. This benefit is generally limited to two to three weeks, although there is no requirement of previous hospitalization. Finally, Part A includes benefits for hospice services for the terminally ill with life expectancies of six months or less. There is a lifetime limit of 210 days in this policy and an annual ceiling on per-enrollee expenditures. Institutional expenses other than those just described are not covered under Part A of Medicare, leaving long-term care as a glaring omission from this program.

Part B of Medicare, which is optional for the elderly (most do purchase it), is designed to cover major medical expenses not incurred as an inpatient in hospitals or other health care institutions. Participants in the program pay a monthly premium for these benefits, set at $28.60 in 1991. In addition, a deductible must be paid and beneficiaries are responsible for a coinsurance payment of 20 percent of the "reasonable charge." Finally, if the physician has not agreed to accept Medicare reimbursement as payment in full, the enrollee is liable for the difference between the actual charges and Medicare reimbursement. This provision was modified slightly in 1991 to say that physicians are limited in how much they can charge Medicare patients in addition to what they receive in reimbursement from the Medicare program. In 1993, the limit will be a total reimbursement (Medicare plus individual) of 115 percent of Medicare-allowed charges. Medicare also covers a variety of "medical and other health services," specifically:

outpatient hospital services
diagnostic laboratory and X-ray services
therapeutic radiology services
outpatient occupational and physical therapy
rural health clinic services
services of clinical psychologists
kidney dialysis services
immunosuppressive drugs furnished in the first year following a Medicare-
    covered transplant procedure
durable medical equipment
services of registered nurse anesthetists
services of physician assistants in certain settings
services in ambulatory surgical centers (Koitz, Reuter, and Merlis 1989).

Services not covered include routine physical checkups, routine dental care, routine foot care, and services considered to be "experimental." Until the last two years, Medicare did not pay for mammography for women, and prescription drugs are still excluded from benefits. Many of the "Medigap" policies sold on the market concentrate on reimbursing the difference between Medicare amounts and actual charges for those services covered by Medicare; they do not address the problem of paying for uncovered services such as long-term care and prescription medications.

Illnesses suffered by the elderly are often exactly those for which expenses are incurred in two of the major uncovered categories—long-term care and prescription medications. The director of the National Institute on Aging has described these examples:

> Alzheimer's disease, osteoporosis, heart disease and stroke predominate among the many diseases that cause chronic disability among the elderly. These conditions bring both physical and emotional pain as people experience and relatives watch a decline in the ability to do things that most of us take for granted. Long-term care is the help needed to cope, and sometimes to survive, when physical or mental disabilities impair the capacity to perform the basic activities of every day life, such as eating, toileting, bathing, dressing and moving about (Williams 1988).

The burden of payment for long-term care actually falls on the state governments through the Medicaid program. After the elderly have exhausted their personal resources during a long-term care stay (and given an average monthly expenditure exceeding $2,500—the Pepper Commission 1990—it may not take long to do so), they become eligible for, and receive, Medicaid benefits, which finance the long-term care stay. As of 1987, Medicaid was paying about 44 percent of the $40.6 billion collected by nursing homes each year (Rovner 1990). For the elderly who do not receive Medicaid benefits, the burden of financing nursing home care is tremendous. One elderly spouse of a man with Alzheimer's disease does not buy meat unless it is marked down near the expiration of the sale date, wears shoes that are over twenty years old, and leaves the air conditioning off until the temperature exceeds 90 degrees (Pepper Commission 1990, 101). In spite of Medicare, the elderly are left without adequate health care coverage.

THE FISCAL BURDEN OF MEDICARE

Looking to the Medicare program for help in resolving the health care access needs of the elderly poses an interesting dilemma for policymakers. Even though it is financed by a growing revenue base, the payroll tax, Medicare's expenditures threaten to outpace revenues. Between 1970 and 1988, Medicare expenditures increased 15.13 percent annually, compared to a 10.96 percent increase for national health expenditures, a 9.87 percent increase in federal outlays, and a 6.39 percent increase in the consumer price index. Between 1975 and 1988, the program grew from 3.9 to 7.4 percent of all federal outlays (Koitz, Reuter, and Merlis 1989). As such a large consumer of federal outlays, Medicare has become a prime target for reductions during budget deliberations in recent years.

In addition to being a part of the annual discussions of how to reduce the federal deficit, the Medicare program is the subject of separate discussions concerning its own future fiscal health. Although the date by which the Health Insurance Trust Fund that finances Medicare Part A and a portion of Part B will be in deficit changes because of changing reimbursement policies, there is widespread agreement that unless action is taken, at some point in the year 2000 it will be in deficit (Long 1985). Since this fear first surfaced in the early 1980s, Congress has taken steps to curb Medicare spending, including enacting the prospective payment system for hospitals and the soon-to-be-phased-in resource-based system to pay physicians. These policy decisions have been designed to meet the objective of reducing the Medicare program's projected expenditures, which means that in this environment it is all the more difficult to suggest increasing the benefits offered by the Medicare program.

POLICY INITIATIVE FOILED: THE MEDICARE CATASTROPHIC ACT

In 1988 Congress was primed to act with a major revision of the Medicare program to extend benefits to the elderly in long-term care, hospitalization, primary care, and prescription medications. The secretary of Health and Human Services, Otis R. Bowen, himself a family practitioner, suggested and supported a major expansion of the Medicare program. With the help of this important Reagan administration official and his staff, Congress fashioned legislation that accomplished the objectives of assuring greater financial access to care. The action on this legislation illustrates the importance of a favorable policy environment, a specific idea, support in the issue network, and particular policy entrepreneurs all coming together to produce dramatic policy change. The environment in 1988 was that of increasing out-of-pocket expenditures for the elderly, and the idea was to change Medicare benefits to reduce that burden. The issue network in Congress was strongly supportive, and with Otis Bowen as a policy entrepreneur, the final piece for success in obtaining legislative change was in place.

The Medicare Catastrophic Coverage Act of 1988 was signed into law on 1 July 1988 and was celebrated as a great policy victory both in Congress and in the Department of Health and Human Services. Its new benefits included unlimited hospitalization without cost after the initial deductible, a ceiling of $1,400 on out-of-pocket expenses for doctor bills (assuming the bills are within the fees allowed by Medicare), payment for prescription drugs after a $600 deductible, an increase to 150 days a year in skilled nursing home care (without a requirement for previous hospitalization), removal of the limit on hospice care, breast cancer screening, and respite benefits for families caring for the infirm elderly. By one estimate, these new benefits would increase Medicare payments to 20 percent of Medicare beneficiaries (Iglehart 1989a).

Enacted in an environment favoring only those new programs that are budget neutral, this dramatic expansion of Medicare benefits was to be financed without increasing the federal deficit. This was accomplished by increasing monthly premiums in the program, by $4 initially and to $10.20 by 1993. In addition, income-related premiums would be paid by the two-fifths of enrollees with the highest incomes. This supplemental premium was limited to $800 per year for an individual and $1,600 for a couple; ten percent of enrollees were expected to pay these maximums (Iglehart 1989a). In discussing these provisions, Iglehart offered this rather prophetic observation: "An estimated 10 percent of enrollees will pay these maximal amounts in 1989, but they represent some of the most articulate members of the elderly, who may be in a position to press their case before the government" (Iglehart 1989a, 334).

Almost immediately after the act was signed into law, a widespread campaign began to repeal its provisions. The campaign was based on the increased premiums being charged to Medicare enrollees, with some, including the Committee to Preserve Social Security and Medicare, implying supreme injustice: "Your Federal Taxes for 1989 May Increase by up to $1,600 ($800 for Singles)—Just Because You Are over the Age of 65!" (Hosenball 1989). An extensive direct mail campaign to the elderly and the subsequent pressure the elderly put on their Congressional representatives was effective. On 29 November 1989 most of the provisions of the act were repealed, retaining breast screening and provisions related to Medicaid (Rovner 1989). Mammography screening was restored as a Medicare benefit in the 1991 Omnibus Budget Reconciliation Act.

Was the repeal of the Medicare Catastrophic Act a signal that major change in federal programs is not possible? Such an interpretation would be extending the Medicare experience to all programs. Not all programs are subject to the lobbying power of the elderly, however. When the intended beneficiaries of new programs form a vocal opposition, we should not expect continued congressional support. The circumstances of this brief legislative history were the result of Congress's efforts to make the new benefits budget neutral. The fiscal constraint will continue to plague future policy initiatives, which would lead to the prediction that any more suggestions for expanded programs will need to be financed by broad-based revenue sources that do not target particular groups. The legislative history of the Medicare Catastrophic Act demonstrates the need to consider policy ideas in the context of the policy environment and the relative influence of various members of the issue network. In this case, the environment seemed to encourage action, but within the issue network, powerful members were opposed to specific features of the policy design.

Along with changes in the roles of actors in the issue network, this case history illustrates an important point about the substance of policy change. When the change was presented to the elderly as one that would increase benefits, support for the act was overwhelming. When the attention focused on the costs of the new program, however, opposition grew. The changing face of the issues can be traced by observing changes in how the nation's media portrayed the legislation. In this case, at least, the media became a player in the issue network by mobilizing public opinion, which in turn influenced members of Congress to repeal the act (Fan and Norem 1992). Initiating and enacting changes in public policies are never a simple matter, since both the general policy environment and the composition of the issue network may change during the design of policies. Such was the case with catastrophic-care legislation.

FURTHER OPTIONS FOR THE ELDERLY

Without the Medicare Catastrophic Act we are still left with the problems of access to care for the elderly. Congress has retreated to smaller, traditionally incremental steps to act on this problem. Representative Stark, one of the key players in the issue network, has introduced the Medigap Reform Act to regulate more thoroughly the nature of supplemental insurance plans sold to the elderly, setting national standards and ending sales of duplicate policies (Cooper

1990). Congress has also expressed a willingness to consider certain specific benefits, such as breast cancer screening (1991 provisions), pap smears (1990 provisions), and home health benefits, but little else.

There may be some hope for the elderly in activities at the state level, combined with private initiatives in long-term care insurance. State governments are considering modifications in the Medicaid program that help the elderly avoid bankruptcy as a result of nursing home expenses. One approach in this effort is to not force the elderly to use all of their private coverage before becoming eligible for Medicaid benefits. Eight states, with planning grants from the Robert Wood Johnson Foundation, are exploring this option: Connecticut, New York, California, Indiana, Massachusetts, New Jersey, Oregon, and Wisconsin (Harnett 1990). Another approach the states can take is to develop long-term care policies for their own employees that can serve as models for others to adopt, which is being done in Alaska, Ohio, and South Carolina (Rovner 1990).

The plight of the near-poor elderly not eligible for Medicaid benefits remains an access-to-care issue. Unfortunately for those persons, they are not as vocal as the politically astute elderly. Therefore, when programs are discussed to resolve financial access problems, the target group remains those under age sixty-five, and the assumption is that Medicare is available and comprehensive to meet the needs of the elderly. This is an issue area in which the members of the issue network will need to prepare more analysis and specific policy suggestions in advance of the time when catastrophic care again emerges on an institutional agenda for action.

Access Problems for Rural Residents

Delivery of health care services in rural communities has always posed problems of how to make advanced medical care available to residents of sparsely settled areas. The problem became more acute in the 1970s and 1980s as the nation's population was more concentrated in urban areas. (There was some return to rural communities in the late 1970s and early 1980s, but the trend reversed and by 1990 was well established as a rural-to-urban movement.) Rural health care issues have been a hot item on the policy agenda since the advent of Medicare's prospective payment system in 1983. That system succeeded in reducing Medicare expenditures for hospital care but perhaps at the expense of forcing some rural hospitals to close and placing many others in financial jeopardy. The issue of losing rural hospitals galvanized a political constituency, represented by, among others, the National Rural Health Association and the Sec-

Small and Rural Hospitals of the American Hospital Association. Rural advocates have pressed for public policies to assist rural hospitals, provide an adequate number of health professionals, and meet special needs such as long-term care for the elderly and emergency medical services for the injured.

The following discussion of rural health care issues provides an opportunity to examine the importance of the implementation of national policies, specifically the new system for reimbursing hospitals, in a federal system in which state governments play an important role, in this case licensing hospitals. The discussion of rural issues also highlights once again the incremental nature of public policy activities and the role for analysis in developing policy alternatives. There is less likelihood for radical change in this area than in most others discussed in this book, primarily because ideas for radical change are not yet well developed. We are edging closer to opportunities for radical restructuring of the delivery system, however, thanks to growing recognition of the inadequacies of the present system.

Discussing the problems in health care delivery in rural communities is a daunting task, since the full array of services to all persons is at issue. The specific policy concerns in recent years have focused on health care facilities, the availability of health care professionals, and services to special populations. In each of these three areas, the most appropriate course of action is one that emphasizes innovative approaches to the delivery of care.

RURAL HEALTH FACILITIES

Hospitals have been the focus of much of the discussion about rural health care: "The rural hospital is the center of the rural health care system" (Rosenblatt and Moscovice 1982). Since the success of the Hill-Burton program, which since 1942 has provided financial assistance to build and expand hospitals throughout the country, many rural citizens have had access to acute care hospitals within a very short distance of their homes. An expectation has been created that all citizens will be within a reasonable distance (usually less than thirty-five miles) of a hospital. This expectation may not be realistic in a time of declining rural populations and reduced payment for inpatient hospital services. Between 1986 and 1989, 120 rural hospitals closed. Although these closures have yet to cause serious problems in accessing health care (because other rural hospitals were nearby), access could be threatened if the trend of closures were to continue.

Rural hospitals are generally small and depend upon a few major resources to sustain themselves financially. Over 70 percent of these institutions contain less than 100 beds (American Hospital Association 1987). They "offer a core of basic services to the populations they serve; emergency, obstetric, and newborn services are virtually ubiquitous in rural hospitals of all sizes" (Hart, Rosenblatt, and Amundson 1989). Rural hospitals are more dependent than their urban counterparts upon public sources for revenue. Approximately 65 percent of rural hospitals receive over 50 percent of their net revenues from public sources, compared to 51 percent of all hospitals. Eleven percent of total revenues for rural hospitals is from Medicare patients, and for hospitals with less than 25 beds the share is 13 percent (American Hospital Association, 1988).

Small rural hospitals have the greatest percentage of Medicare patients of any grouping of hospitals, with over 40 percent of their patients being financed by Medicare (Mick and Morlock 1990). Rural hospitals experience a higher burden in providing care that is not paid for by others, showing 5.49 percent bad debt and charity care compared to 4.89 percent for urban hospitals in 1988 (Mick and Morlock 1990). These data indicate that it is very difficult for rural hospitals to shift their costs among payers when one major source demands lower reimbursements, as has been the case with Medicare since 1983. There are fewer opportunities for cost shifting because of the higher percentage of patients who are Medicare clients and the higher debt burden in rural hospitals.

When the prospective payment system (PPS) began, rural hospitals were reimbursed lesser amounts than urban hospitals for the same services. The resulting payments to rural hospitals were not sufficient to reimburse all costs for the cases treated; operating margins for rural hospitals in PPS were negative in the fourth and fifth years (1987 and 1988), with rural hospitals under 100 beds suffering the worst (margins of −3.5 percent for those under 50 beds and −4.0 percent for those between 50 and 100 beds) (OTA 1990).

Negative operating margins from a single payer may not be a problem, assuming one of the following two conditions: (1) costs can be shifted to other revenue sources, or (2) the negative margins are only a temporary phenomenon. For many rural hospitals, neither of those conditions holds. First, the high percentage of revenue from Medicare for the average rural hospital disguises the reality that for some rural hospitals the percent of Medicare patients exceeds 75 (research findings from my survey of hospital administrators in six midwestern states). Second, negative operating margins have affected many rural hospitals for at least the past three years, and they show few signs of improving. That being the case, hospitals that had cash reserves that permitted surviving short-term cash flow problems cannot support indefinitely the presence of negative operating margins.

Two policy issues are implicit in discussing the problems of rural hospitals. First, what can be done to relieve essential (for access) rural hospitals of their fiscal strain? Second, what are the options for communities in which rural hospitals are closing?

Congress has been actively seeking legislative remedies for the problems facing rural hospitals, especially since the formation of the Senate Rural Health Caucus in 1986 and the House of Representatives Rural Health Care Coalition in 1987. Even the legislation establishing PPS recognized the need for special consideration of some rural hospitals, creating special classifications and reimbursement policies for sole community-provider hospitals (generally more than thirty-five to fifty miles from the nearest full-service hospital) and rural referral centers (generally large hospitals that receive transfers from other, smaller rural hospitals). One area of policy adjustment after 1983, and especially after 1987, was to expand the eligibility for designation as a sole community-provider hospital, which permitted more hospitals to be reimbursed on their own hospital's cost experience rather than on the average costs used to calculate reimbursement under PPS.

Changes affecting Medicare payment to rural hospitals have been enacted as provisions in omnibus budget reconciliation acts, beginning in 1986. These have been incremental changes, sometimes technical in nature, which have provided more opportunities for rural hospitals to improve their finances by increasing revenues from Medicare. The changes indicate the detailed work at least some members of Congress and their staffs are willing to undertake in order to change public policy. Further, the vehicle of an omnibus bill that is enacted every year has been used extensively by members of the health care issue network.

In the Omnibus Budget Reconciliation Act (OBRA) of 1986, Congress began to address the particular problems of rural hospitals with three important provisions. They separated the urban and rural pools of funds used to pay for *outliers,* those cases in which excessive expenditures above the PPS allotment are incurred (this ended the practice of using revenues otherwise intended for rural hospitals to reimburse expensive cases in urban hospitals). They provided early payments to hospitals with fewer than one hundred beds. And they changed the criteria for rural referral centers to allow more hospitals to qualify.

The OBRA of 1987 included provisions that: increased the payment for rural hospitals more than the increase for urban hospitals; allowed rural hospitals located adjacent to metropolitan statistical areas to be defined as urban hospitals; expanded the swing-bed program (permits using the same beds as acute care and long-term care—the latter increases hospital revenues) to include hospitals with under one hundred beds (from under fifty beds); authorized a rural health care transition program to provide assistance to hospitals and others wishing to adopt new service delivery strategies; required a report on the appropriateness of separate urban and rural rates; and authorized small rural hospitals to serve as residency training sites for physicians (Patton 1988).

In the last two reconciliation bills, Congress has included provisions that: appropriate funds for the rural health care transition program, phase out the differential between urban and rural hospital reimbursement under PPS, and establish a program to create two new categories of rural hospitals (essential access hospitals and primary care hospitals) that would be part of regional networks to assure the availability of essential care without requiring all hospitals to provide the full array of services.

These incremental actions of Congress have helped to level the playing field in reimbursement to rural hospitals vis-à-vis all other hospitals. That level of assistance, however, may not be sufficient to sustain rural hospitals, since much of their problem is a result of low overall occupancy (less than 50 percent of the beds in many rural hospitals are filled at any given time). To the extent Congress wants to guarantee the financial survival of rural hospitals, more radical policies may be needed that simply provide the funding necessary to keep those facilities operating. On the other hand, national policy could be used to provide incentives to hospitals and communities to reconfigure health care delivery and use the hospital facilities in ways different from the current practices.

The problems confronting rural hospitals are not ones that require nonincremental policies. Instead, current trends toward changes in hospital services are sufficient to resolve the problems for most of these hospitals. Although some of those changes may seem radical (such as the medical assistance facilities in Montana that will become hospitals that provide very limited care), they are not complete departures from present practices. A dramatic departure would resemble an abandonment of health care delivery in rural communities or a publicly imposed reconfiguration of all health care services in a large geographic region (several counties).

Many rural hospitals achieve success in today's fiscal environment by adopting any of a number of management strategies. One of the most common of those is diversifying services, adding such programs as nursing home care, home health care, birthing centers, or psychiatric facilities. The most common new program is to add an organized outpatient department to the hospital, as 416 rural hospitals did between 1982 and 1985 (Ermann 1990). Outpatient revenues rose from 14 percent of all gross patient revenues to 18 percent between 1983 and 1985 (Ermann 1990). This particular diversification generates revenue not constrained by PPS and may help attract persons to the hospital who need simple procedures. Another very common diversification strategy is to establish a home health care program to serve the elderly, who represent a larger percentage of rural populations than they do in urban areas. These programs are more difficult to establish, given the dispersion of rural population, but have been used successfully in many hospitals.

A strategy that has gained popularity since more rural hospitals have closed has been to establish satellite and specialty clinics. These clinics generate revenues for the home institution, at the same time extending medical care services to a community otherwise underserved. Two other strategies are seeing increased use, especially with the advent of transition grants from the federal government. The first of those is downsizing, which means delicensing hospital beds and reducing the number of employees. The new federal program to establish primary care hospitals also encourages downsizing. The second strategy is to engage in more targeted and aggressive marketing: "A 1986 AHA survey of 500 small, rural hospitals revealed that 27 percent of responding institutions increased their marketing budgets 5 percent or more from 1985 to 1986" (Ermann 1990, 60). A final approach is to form alliances among several rural hospitals, and possibly with urban affiliates, to lower costs for supplies and materials, and to specialize among the hospitals belonging to the alliance. The Robert Wood Johnson Foundation is currently sponsoring thirteen efforts to establish rural hospital consortia (Christianson et. al. 1990).

Rural hospitals can succeed, although there is reason to believe that many more may fail in the next decade. Just as the average patient revenue margin disguises some big losers since PPS, it also disguises some big winners among rural hospitals. The most important steps taken in public policy have been to create incentives for innovative action and management in rural hospitals, and policies that remove any existing regulatory barriers to appropriate experimentation. Regulations are necessary to assure the quality of care in all hospitals, but the regulations that force hospitals to offer services not sustainable in rural environments must be removed, an action being taken by state governments.

ACCESS TO HEALTH PERSONNEL IN RURAL AREAS

The prognosis for maintaining reasonable numbers of health professionals in rural areas is not as bright as the one for hospitals. Rural America is plagued by a shortage of trained medical personnel in all professions, from primary care physicians to nurse midwives, from psychiatrists to social workers, and from surgeons to nurse anesthetists. Although there is potential for some innovations that would lessen the requirements for physicians in all rural areas, there is not the same flexibility as there is in the case of rural hospitals. There are several initiatives under way in various states to help resolve the problem of personnel shortages, but nothing short of a major public policy commitment can resolve this problem.

The number of active physicians per 100,000 residents in rural areas is less than half that in urban areas. Lest we think that may be good, given what may be perceived to be a surplus of physicians in urban areas, we should realize that in 1988 there were 111 rural counties (with a total population of 325,100) with no physician (OTA 1990). The shortage of physicians is even more severe if we focus on primary care physicians. These professionals are especially important in rural medicine, since there are fewer specialists available. The ratio of primary care physicians per 100,000 persons in 1988 was 87 in metropolitan counties, 55 in rural counties, and 47 in frontier (less than six persons per square mile) counties. There were 176 rural counties with no primary care physicians, with a total of 713,700 persons (Summer 1991). We cannot look to a growth in the number of physicians to resolve these shortages, for three reasons. First, the general supply of primary care physicians is increasing more slowly in rural than in urban areas (OTA 1990). Second, physicians already located in rural areas are leaving. A large number of them are nearing retirement age (13 percent of rural physicians are age sixty-five and over, compared to 9 percent in urban areas). Third, younger physicians may be leaving the rural counties as a matter of professional preference—one survey in 1988 found that 26 percent of the responding rural physicians anticipated leaving within five years (OTA 1990).

There are also needs to increase the availability of professionals in practices other than general and family practice. In 1988, almost two-thirds of all nonmetropolitan counties had no pediatricians, and the number of pediatricians per 100,000 women of childbearing age was 22.3 in rural counties, compared to 69.7 in metropolitan counties (Summer 1991). Midlevel health professionals are also in short supply, and their skills could help in counties experiencing physician shortages. In recent years, metropolitan settings have become increasingly enticing to nurse practitioners and physicians' assistants because of better preparation for specialized practices in large urban hospitals (OTA 1990). The percentage of physicians' assistants in primary care practice declined from 75 percent in 1978 to 65 percent in 1986, and the percent practicing in small communities (less than 10,000 residents) declined from 27 percent in 1981 to 20 percent in 1990 (OTA 1990). The same pattern holds for nurse-midwives and certified registered nurse anesthetists. Finally, the nursing shortage of the late 1980s has left rural communities in more critical condition than urban areas.

Shortages of personnel translate into access problems for rural residents. The federal government designates certain areas as health manpower shortage areas (HMSAS), based on having a population-to-primary care physician ratio of at least 3,500:1 and being an area adjacent to others in which primary medical care personnel are overused. By that definition, 67 percent of the HMSAS in 1988 were in rural areas, and 29 percent of the rural population live in HMSAS, compared to 9 percent of the urban population (OTA 1990).

There are very few short-term options available to resolve the personnel shortages in rural areas. Clearly, more professionals are needed. Training those professionals, however, requires several years, and the rural communities must still compete with urban areas for the services of those professionals. During the early and mid-1980s, an assumption gained favor that a general increase in the supply of medical personnel would have the effect of leveling the distribution of health professionals across specialties and geographic areas. Caught up in that optimism, the federal government discontinued its direct involvement of providing financial assistance to medical students in return for a commitment to practice in shortage areas, the National Health Service Corps. Appropriations for that program fell from $153.6 million in 1980 to $38.8 million in 1988 (Summer 1991). In fact, the program limped from 1988 to 1990 without being reauthorized. In 1990, though, Congress was once again convinced of the need for an aggressive federal program. The members of the issue network, particularly state and local officials and the National Rural Health Association, worked hard to present analysis to key members of Congress that serious shortages of health care professionals not only continued but were growing. The 1990 legislation reestablished a scholarship program, continued a loan repayment program, and reauthorized grants to states providing loan programs. Further, the new act includes provisions designed to improve the effectiveness of the program. In particular, priorities are given to students from disadvantaged backgrounds, counseling is provided to scholarship recipients to prepare them to practice in underserved areas, priority in placement is given to areas in which primary health services are coordinated with social and health services, and exchange programs with teaching centers are established (Summer 1991).

Providing funding for the National Health Service Corps is a major step toward redressing the problem of personnel shortages in rural areas, but more will be needed. The corps only affects the percent of graduating physicians practicing in shortage areas, and then only for a limited period of time for each student. Additional programs are needed that increase the total supply of physicians and create incentives for permanent practice in rural areas. As is so often the case in our federal system, we should look to the states for innovative approaches to meet these two needs. For example, in Washington, components of medical education are decentralized to rural locations in four states (Washington, Idaho, Montana, and Alaska), and 23 percent of graduates from that program practice in rural areas (compared to 13 percent of all U.S. physicians); 61 percent were in primary care practice, compared to 35 percent of all U.S. physicians (OTA 1990). The University of Minnesota has a program providing a nine- to twelve-month rural clinical preceptorship for third-year medical students, and 57 percent of the former students in that program are practicing in rural areas (OTA 1990). Other states, including South Dakota and Nebraska, have established telecommunications systems to link rural physicians with university-based services in metropolitan areas (OTA 1990). In Oregon, physicians and other health professionals practicing in rural areas are allowed income tax credits of up to $5,000 (McCloskey and Leuhrs 1990).

Health personnel policies adopted to date focus on recruiting and retaining physicians in rural communities. But there have not been any comprehensive policies that attempt to recruit and retain a mixture of health care professionals most appropriate in a rural health care delivery system. Perhaps it is too much to hope for such a comprehensive policy development, just as it is to hope for national health insurance. Although there has been a great deal of attention to the health needs of rural communities, the concern of what to do about rural hospitals and physicians seems to overshadow all else, especially in national developments.

SPECIAL RURAL POPULATIONS:
THE MENTALLY ILL, THE ELDERLY, AND PREGNANT WOMEN

Another problem receiving only minimal public policy attention to date is that of delivering services to rural residents with mental health problems. In recent years researchers have found the prevalence of mental health problems among rural residents higher than previously known. During and following the farm crisis of the early 1980s, interest increased in knowing more about the mental problems of rural residents and how they coped with those problems. One study found higher rates of alcohol abuse and/or dependence, and cognitive deficit in rural areas (Blazer et al. 1985). In a study of the effects of the farm crisis, Beeson and Johnson (1987) found that the rate of depression in farm communities increased from 11 percent in 1981 to 21 percent in 1986. Mental health centers located in rural areas reported significant increases in the numbers of clients during the years of the farm crisis (Wagenfeld 1990; Murray and Keller 1991).

The health care delivery system in rural areas is not well-equipped to deal with problems related to mental health. These areas rely on mental health clinics that serve large areas: "A typical rural mental health service delivery areas is 5,000 square miles, and the largest such area covers more than 60,000 square miles" (Murray and Keller 1991, 224). Further, existing Community Mental Health Centers have not always been responsive to the particular problems of rural residents (Wagenfeld 1990). More success may be realized by providing mental health services in the context of general health care services in the offices of primary care physicians (Wagenfeld 1990). Innovative approaches to the delivery of mental health services that take advantage of natural points of contact with rural residents seem to offer the best hope for treating this problem (Murray and Keller 1991). Even that approach, however, will require training in mental health counseling and more mental health professionals, both of which are in short supply in rural areas. The cultural environment in which mental health problems arise is much different in rural areas, and the appropriate responses to those problems will necessarily also be different from the traditional urban models. Only after this issue becomes a higher priority on the public policy agenda, however, would such changes be expected. Reimbursement policies and training incentives are needed that would encourage an appropriate response to the needs of rural residents.

A discussion of particular populations with special unmet needs in rural areas could continue at great length. Two groups in particular stand out. The first of those is the elderly. The percentage of persons age sixty-five and over is higher in rural counties than in urban counties, and their health care needs are not different. The rural elderly develop needs for custodial care (meals, help in cleaning, and other activities of daily living) that could be met either through an array of community services or through placement in a nursing home. In rural communities, the former are difficult to provide because of problems of economies of scale, leading to what is an inappropriately high rate of placement in nursing homes. More needs to be done to care for the elderly in the environment most appropriate for them.

Another group warranting special attention is pregnant women. Infant mortality rates are unacceptably high in many rural counties, higher in some than in third-world nations (Hughes and Rosenbaum 1989). There are special problems in attracting the appropriate health professionals to rural communities to provide proper prenatal care for expectant mothers, and there are problems in financing those services since in many of these counties the rate of the uninsured is also higher than typical for the nation (Hughes and Rosenbaum 1989). Policies are needed to address both the health personnel and the finance issues. Finally, there are special problems related to the nature of rural communities and the desire of young women not to reveal pregnancy until it is obvious. That desire is more easily accommodated in urban areas with enclaves of anonymity than in small rural communities. This is another area, similar to mental health, in which adopting models tailored specifically to the needs of rural communities is important.

ACCESS AS A RURAL ISSUE SUMMARIZED

Residents of rural areas experience difficulties accessing the full array of health care services. Policy responses to date have focused on one dimension of the health care delivery system at a time, with particular attention on hospitals and physicians. Although these two components of the system have traditionally been considered the building blocks of health care, they are not always the most appropriate focus in remote rural areas.

Local and regional approaches to providing health care in rural areas should include models that match health care providers with community needs and resources. This philosophy would mean that very small communities (less than 1,500 residents) are unlikely to have either hospitals or physicians. Instead they could be served by clinics staffed by midlevel medical practitioners. Larger communities could be served by limited service hospitals (similar to the Montana medical assistance facilities). The largest communities would have full-service hospitals, physicians, and a limited number of specialists. A scheme for organizing rural health care might parallel the Rural Heath Care System presented by Hart (1988). A series of environmental variables (political, regulatory, technological, personnel, financial, economic, epidemiological, and demographic) are matched with the settings for service delivery (environmental, ambulatory, transport, residential, inpatient) and ownership status (for-profit, not-for-profit, and public) to create the health care system best suited for particular areas. The task for public policymakers is to facilitate, and, if necessary, force the health care delivery system to make the appropriate changes in rural areas. In the short run, crises in particular communities losing hospitals and physicians will continue to dominate the policy agenda, but eventually the broader discussion will ensue and policies will be considered. These policies will be the product of actions in the federal system; that is, the local solutions will be developed by state and local units of government with national support and incentives.

Other Issues in Access to Care

Problems of obtaining health care occur for many groups in our society not discussed at length in this chapter. For example, access to prenatal care is a problem for expectant mothers in cities as well as in rural areas. There are inner cities in this nation with infant mortality rates exceeding those found in third-world countries. Access for the mentally ill in metropolitan areas is also a problem, particularly the full array of services those individuals should use. Deinstitutionalizing the mentally ill in recent years has created problems because local communities have not always been prepared with alternative forms of treatment and housing for those individuals.

There are other populations with problems of limited access. Four of them are described in the following pages: low-income mothers and children, persons with acquired immune deficiency syndrome (AIDS), elderly needing long-term-care services, and minorities. Each of these groups warrants full consideration in debates focused on reforming the health care delivery system to improve access. The general context of the debate, though, is the same: balancing demands for improved access with those to restrain health expenditures and yet provide the best possible care.

LOW-INCOME MOTHERS AND CHILDREN

Low-income mothers and their children have problems accessing the health care system both because they lack insurance and because they generally live in medically underserved areas. Limited access among pregnant women explains, at least in part, the poor performance of the United States's birth data compared with those of other nations. Limited access among children creates problems of untreated chronic health conditions that in turn lead both to increased medical expenditures and to loss of productivity to society.

Between 1977 and 1987, the percentage of children with private health insurance benefits declined considerably, from 73.6 percent to 67.6 percent (Cunningham and Monheit 1990). Data from the national medical expenditure surveys of those years also show an increase in the percentage of children receiving Medicaid benefits, from 13.6 to 14.6 percent, and in those without any health insurance, from 12.7 to 17.89 percent (Cunningham and Monheit, 1990). Even more dramatic changes in the health insurance status of poor children occurred during those years (see table 5.4).

In recent years Congress has acted to improve the availability of health insurance for children. Several initiatives to expand access to Medicaid were described earlier in this chapter. As of 1991, all children below the age of eight in families with incomes below the federal poverty guidelines are eligible for Medicaid benefits. By 2001, all children under age nineteen in families with incomes below the federal poverty guidelines will be eligible. All children may also be the beneficiaries of a new tax policy that permits low-income families to obtain a tax credit for purchasing health insurance for children. The credit is limited to no more than 6 percent of taxable income and cannot exceed the cost of the insurance premium for the child. These policy changes represent important efforts to expand access to care for children, but they are not sufficient to do so.

Earlier in this chapter the problems of rural areas in attracting and retaining an adequate supply of health professionals were documented. Much the same situation exists in many of the nation's inner cities. A study of health care for children in Chicago, for example, concluded that new policies expanding eligibility for the financial benefits of Medicaid will have very little impact on access. The greater problem for poor children in Chicago is access to health professionals. The study's authors suggest that devoting resources to institutions to provide services would have a greater impact on care for poor children than does expanding eligibility for Medicaid (Fossett et al. 1992).

Low-income mothers face the same problems as their children in accessing medical services. Pregnant women in low-income families are far less likely to receive health services during their pregnancies than are women in other income categories. Once again, the reaction of policymakers has been to incrementally change the existing Medicaid program by requiring that all pregnant women in families with incomes below the federal poverty guidelines be eligible for Medicaid benefits. That federal mandate, however, did not increase appropriations so that more providers might participate in the Medicaid program

Table 5.4 Health Insurance Status of Children, 1977 and 1987

Year	Income Level	Privately Insured (%)	Public Insurance (%)	No Insurance (%)
1977	Below poverty	27.6	50.3	21.8
	100–199% of poverty	62.0	16.9	20.9
1987	Below poverty	26.3	37.6	36.0
	100–199% of poverty	49.3	23.7	27.0

Source: Cunningham and Monheit (1990), exhibit 3, p.83.

to handle the anticipated increase in the number of clients. In many states, less than 60 percent of physicians participate in the Medicaid program, and often the reason for nonparticipation is the level of payment for services. In 1983, only 53 percent of pediatricians in the country accepted Medicaid patients; that low percentage is thought to be true as of 1990 (Sardell 1990). In 1987 a survey of women in the Medicaid program revealed the following reasons for not accessing prenatal care: financial problems, transportation, time conflicts, ambivalent feelings, belief that care is not important, and lack of knowledge (Schlesinger and Kronebusch 1990).

Generating interest in the health care problems of children is easy in our political system and there is little resistance to doing something to provide access to care. Policies to date, however, have been only incremental changes to financial eligibility for services and have not addressed other pressing problems. Absent changes in the delivery system that redistributes resources, poor mothers and their children will continue to experience problems accessing health care services.

PERSONS WITH AIDS

Persons with AIDS, those who have progressed from infection by HIV to actually having the disease and therefore needing more expensive treatment, also have problems obtaining health care. Persons with this disease experience difficulty obtaining insurance coverage, and their illness leads to catastrophic health care expenditures. The average cost of treating a person with AIDS is estimated to be $32,000 per year, of which $24,000 is for hospital services (Hellinger 1991). Financial access can be a barrier, particularly for persons without adequate health insurance benefits. Such is the case for many persons with AIDS, particularly homosexual men. A survey of that population in two large cities found that persons with AIDS were less likely to have private health insurance (64 percent versus 90 percent of those without AIDS) and more likely to lose health insurance coverage (10 percent versus 2 percent of patients without AIDS). Finally, persons with AIDS are likely to enroll in Medicaid programs (Kass et al. 1991).

As was the case for children, financial access to services may be the least of the access problems facing persons with AIDS. Just as serious a problem is denial of access by providers. Unfortunately the story of one person who was not allowed to see two different dentists because of the fear of spreading the infection is not atypical (National Commission on Acquired Immune Deficiency Syndrome 1991). In some local areas, providing treatment to AIDS patients may strain systems already serving as the principal providers to patients with limited ability to pay. Such has been the case in New York City hospitals.

The AIDS epidemic presents a special challenge to policymakers committed to universal access to health care services. The services required are expensive, and the population in need is relatively small. Further, the care is to patients who are terminally ill. Serious questions of cost-effectiveness arise in any discussion of treatment for persons with AIDS. Providing access to that group may strain the system's abilities to provide access to others.

LONG-TERM CARE

Earlier in this chapter, I discussed at some length the health care needs of the elderly. That discussion, though, did not include one final access issue for that age group, long-term care. The most frail of the elderly population, those unable to care for themselves but not acutely ill, have traditionally been cared for in nursing homes. Because the percentage of the population over age sixty-five, and within that group those over eighty-five, is expected to increase dramatically after the turn of the century, assuring access to long-term care is becoming an increasingly important issue in public policy.

As was the case in considering access for other populations, financial ability to seek care is again a critical concern. In this instance, the problem is financing the nursing home costs, which in most cases will exceed two thousand dollars per month. There are insurance companies that offer special policies with benefits to pay those costs. Only a very small percentage of the elderly, however, are purchasing long-term care insurance. As of 1990, only 5 percent of the elderly had done so (Cohen, Kuman, and Wallack 1992). Most of the elderly begin their nursing home stays paying for the services themselves but then change to Medicaid after their personal resources are spent. In 1987, approximately 61 percent of nursing home clients were enrolled in the Medicaid program (Farley-Short et al. 1992). Public policy considerations about long-term care focused on the Medicare Catastrophic Coverage Act of 1988, and in Congress activities virtually died with the repeal of that legislation.

Again, just as was the case for other groups, financing care is only part of the access problem for the elderly and long-term care. Just as important, nursing homes in many regions are full, oftentimes with waiting lists for admission. If the number of elderly requiring institutionalization continues to increase, the system will need to grow. The frail elderly, however, do not all require institutionalization. Public policies are affecting this dimension of the access problem. The Medicare program provides coverage for home health services so that clients need not be in a nursing home. It also includes benefits for hospice care for the terminally ill in the final months of their lives. Both measures keep the elderly out of nursing homes. There are many efforts under way to expand community-based services that provide the elderly with meals, homemaking services, financial services, and other assistance with the activities of daily living. As of 1992, however, these programs are few in number and serve only a limited number of clients.

MINORITIES

The last group with access problems that warrants special mention is the minority population of the United States. Hispanics, African Americans, Asian Americans, and Native Americans, to name the most prevalent, all experience special difficulties accessing the health care delivery system. In some instances the interaction of low-income and minority status creates difficulties; in others the interaction of special cultural habits and minority status causes problems in accessing health care. Resolving the problems confronting these groups requires policies designed to encourage professional education programs sensitive to the special needs of minorities and programs to expand the delivery of services to areas populated by minorities (many of which are included in areas with a designated shortage of health care workers).

Conclusion

In a nation where over thirty-three million citizens are without any health insurance coverage, where the public policy designed to serve the elderly does not include long-term care or prescription medicine, and where rural communities are isolated from any medical care professionals, access to basic health care remains a serious problem. Without a public policy of universal health care coverage for all Americans, we are left with a patchwork of efforts to extend essential health care services to those currently without.

Incremental approaches to resolving the problems of access can help address particular problems, but they will not eliminate all barriers to access to health care. Given the political system and current budget problems that plague all levels of government, however, we cannot expect other than incremental approaches in the short term. Expansion of the issue network and increased participation from analytical experts (both in and out of government) should facilitate creative approaches to some of these problems, particularly those not involving direct infusions of money. For example, we should expect more creative approaches to configuring the health care delivery system in rural areas. We should also expect an increased use of alternative modes of health care delivery for the elderly. Finally, we should expect to see increased diversification in the education system so that providers are more prepared to deal with the special problems of the mentally ill and minority populations.

These policies will prove the value of the federal system of government. That is, new programs can be tried in various states, and general suggestions can be shaped within particular communities to meet their particular needs. The use of different types of health care institutions to provide care in rural areas, including Montana's medical assistance facilities, is one example of this atmosphere of experimentation. New educational programs that create incentives to practice in rural areas are another.

It may seem odd to say this, but the problems of access being addressed now are treated as new problems. True, there have always been uninsured persons, rural citizens with inadequate care, and minorities with limited access. Policy attention, however, was focused almost exclusively on cost containment issues for over a decade, and access issues were overlooked. Therefore, it is now necessary to build approaches to resolving those problems before we should expect dramatic change. The issues of access are being addressed in the context of the political and fiscal environment of the 1990s, which means solutions are sought that require a minimum of new public resources. Until a new idea catches fire and becomes the dominant approach, we should expect continued incremental adjustments. The winds of change have not yet swept the land demanding radical change to end problems of access to health care.

6

. . .

Issues in
Quality of Health Care

Medical care professionals who care for the sick are licensed by public boards and certified as eligible to be reimbursed by government and other payers. The quality of care delivered by those professionals varies. Public policymakers continue to address issues involving the quality of the medical care provided to American citizens. During the 1970s and 1980s, the context for discussing quality was the cost of assuring redress for inappropriate care. That is, public policy-makers were concerned (and still are) with the cost of malpractice litigation. As the decade of the 1980s drew to a close, discussions of quality of medical care became linked to cost-containment policies. By discovering frequent use of often medically unnecessary procedures (such as hysterectomies), government decision makers hoped to save funds by denying payment for those procedures.

The Health Care Financing Administration (HCFA), U.S. Department of Health and Human Services, initiated efforts to monitor the quality of care provided in hospitals and nursing homes. The HCFA addressed quality issues by supporting research to refine measures of quality and by publishing information about the mortality rates of hospitals. An emphasis on the cost-containment implications of improving the quality of care helped motivate Congress to create the Agency for Health Care Policy and Research (AHCPR) and provide it with millions of dollars to sponsor research establishing the effectiveness (or lack thereof) of medical procedures.

By the 1990s, debates about quality of care expanded to include renewed concern about the quality of care being given to patients and access to the best quality of care for all persons. Research sponsored by the AHCPR related to medical effectiveness, although done in hopes of some reduction in costs of care, has evolved into a program designed to develop and disseminate medical practice guidelines that specify effective courses of action to take when treating certain specific conditions.

Four separate topics will be discussed in addressing issues related to quality of care. First, the "malpractice crisis" is analyzed as an example of how a mechanism designed to help assure quality leads to a cost problem. Second, the effort to develop medical practice guidelines from research on the outcomes of medical procedures is analyzed as an example of adhering to quality-of-care standards that could also contain costs. Third, discussions of rationing health care will be reviewed as an illustration of how redesigning health care delivery and finance might affect the quality of care. Fourth, sustaining a healthy life will be linked to measures that can prevent ill health.

Quality of Care and Malpractice

State and national elected officials have been suggesting and enacting policies to resolve problems of access to, and cost of, medical care attributed to the high cost of malpractice insurance. It would be easy, therefore, to consider this an issue of access or cost containment. The problem originates, however, in a concern about the quality of care delivered by providers, particularly certain specialists, including obstetricians, surgeons, and nurse midwives.

Medical professionals do err, and when errors occur, patients expect some form of redress. For example, when a surgeon in Maryland diverted the wrong section of person's bowel into a colostomy bag, causing severe pain and eventually death, the patient's family appropriately had the recourse of legal action against that physician (*Washington Post* 1988, A17). Although malpractice may not always be linked directly with incompetence among physicians, malpractice claims are a valid indicator of a problem in delivering quality medical care (Waxman 1987).

If malpractice claims were limited in number and size (dollars per claim) a crisis would be unlikely. The number and size of claims increased dramatically in the 1970s and 1980s, however, precipitating a persisting crisis. There are two logical approaches to dealing with the crisis: tighter control over the quality of physicians who practice so there is less reason to initiate malpractice litigation, and/or reform of the legal system to lower aggregate costs of malpractice procedures. These actions can be taken by both the national and the separate state governments.

BREADTH OF THE PROBLEM

Three adverse consequences result from increases in malpractice claims against medical professionals. First, the costs of malpractice insurance increase, and those costs are passed on to consumers. Second, as those costs increase, certain medical specialties are less attractive as career options, which precipitates shortages in those specialties. Third, physicians are more likely to practice defensively, which can include unnecessary procedures or diagnostic tests.

Malpractice insurance premiums for all physicians increased at least 75 percent from 1983 to 1986, and from at least 2.9 percent of physicians' gross revenues to at least 4.0 percent (the exact increase varies by whose survey data are used). Increases were more dramatic for certain specialists: for obstetrics/gynecology the change in payments was 104.7 percent; for radiology 93.0 percent, and for urology 84.1 percent (Rosenbach and Stone 1990). In Florida during 1988, premiums for some doctors were approaching $200,000 per year (*New York Times* 1988).

Premiums are only part of the reason legal activities in malpractice suits increase the costs of health care. Physicians concerned about their potential liability are likely to engage in practice styles that include a number of procedures not immediately necessary for patient welfare. For example, a survey of physicians in Maryland found the most frequent action to avoid malpractice charges was to engage in risk-reduction practices, including adding more diagnostic testing (Weisman et al. 1989). The marginal value of additional testing is questionable, but the value in preempting malpractice litigation may be quite high. Physicians in that survey also reported providing more information to patients, which should benefit both the physician and the patient. They also reported avoiding certain patients and services, which may not have a direct effect on costs but will have an effect on access to care. In a report on national surveys of physicians, 20 percent were said to have changed practice patterns, including adding tests and discontinuing some services such as surgery (Rosenbach and Stone 1990).

Even more serious than the direct effect on costs, increased malpractice activities may precipitate physicians leaving certain specialties and/or not providing certain services. In rural Montana, for example, the costs of malpractice insurance, approximately $65,000 per year, contribute directly to an absence of obstetricians. In rural areas, costs that high are difficult to absorb because of a limited volume of patients. As a result, in Montana during 1987, almost half of the doctors previously delivering babies stopped doing so, and one hospital had to discontinue admitting women for delivery. The nearest institution admitting pregnant women was ninety miles away (Horowitz 1988). Nationally, somewhere between 16 and 49 percent of obstetricians and gynecologists are reducing care to high-risk women because of concern about liability (Rostow, Osterweis, and Bulger 1989).

Shortages of providers may affect more than obstetrical care, as was true in Florida in 1987. Rapidly increasing costs of malpractice insurance for emergency room surgeons led many to refuse to see patients, forcing fifty-seven hospitals to close their emergency rooms (Specter 1987). Other specialists in Florida have also seen premiums increase dramatically, for neurosurgeons from $37,569 in 1983 to $192,420 in 1987 (*New York Times* 1988).

In sum, the frequency and costs of malpractice claims have precipitated a crisis for the delivery of medical care. Premiums for malpractice insurance were the fastest-rising component of physician charges between 1983 and 1989 (Brightbill 1991a). Median jury awards in 1990 were $450,000, and nine hundred medical malpractice lawsuits are filed daily in the United States (Brightbill 1991b). Rates for some specialties such as obstetrics can present disproportionate burdens to those with low volumes of cases, driving them out of the practice entirely. When that occurs, access to care may be denied for some populations.

POLICIES TO RELIEVE THE MALPRACTICE CRISIS

The federal government began its actions to relieve the malpractice crisis and emphasize greater attention to policing the quality of medical care with the Health Care Quality Act of 1986. This legislation mandated the creation of a national data base within the Department of Health and Human Services to provide data on legal actions against health care providers. This information helps people recruiting physicians in one state know of actions against those physicians in other states. Additional national action has been suggested to reform legal proceedings in order to lower the costs of malpractice claims and therefore affect the premiums charged to providers. Senator Orrin Hatch (Republican member of the Committee on Labor and Human Resources) has introduced legislation that would mandate periodic payment of malpractice awards (lowering the costs of paying large sums in one installment), limit awards for economic damage, and set a ceiling on contingency fees collected by attorneys (ending the incentive of securing large awards because the attorney retains a percent of the award) (Brightbill 1991b). Former President George Bush suggested forcing states to reform medical malpractice laws by using the leverage of federal reimbursement polices. In those states without tort reform, Medicare and Medicaid payments would be withheld from hospitals. These specific reforms would have been required in the president's plan: limiting the amount of noneconomic damages, allowing for periodic payment of awards, creating procedures to settle claims out of court, and eliminating the rule forbidding the judge to hear evidence of other sources of payment to the plaintiff (Brightbill 1991a).

As implied by ex-President Bush's suggested policies, state governments have the most direct control over policies influencing the costs and frequencies of malpractice judgments. State responses have been forthcoming, including limiting jury awards for noneconomic damages in ten states to between $250,000 and $500,000. Twenty states have limited or prohibited punitive damages, and some states have even established penalties for frivolous lawsuits (Brightbill 1991b). Reforms of this nature can be effective: malpractice claims fell 30 percent in Connecticut after tort reform in 1986, and the number of cases in Maryland fell nearly 50 percent after frivolous medical lawsuits were limited and noneconomic damages were capped at $350,000 (Brightbill 1991b).

These reforms are encouraging and well advised. The issue remains serious, however, because not all states have taken comprehensive action. We should expect the pressure to reform malpractice statutes to continue until the insurance premiums no longer lead to cost increases or shortages of medical professionals. Although tort reform could help alleviate some of the pressures caused by the increase in malpractice litigation, such measures only attack the symptoms of a greater problem. The problem is, at least in part, evidence of incompetence among a few providers. Overall quality of care suffers and public confidence in the medical profession erodes if inappropriate actions by providers do not lead to disciplinary action. In New York, a step to toughen discipline of physicians was taken in 1975 when the responsibility for bringing disciplinary action was shifted from the Department of Education to the Department of Health (although the Department of Education continues to have some responsibility). More could be done to strengthen the procedures in that state (Lieberman 1987). During 1988, Maryland took steps to toughen its procedures for disciplining physicians by providing funding for additional investigators, creating a new board to regulate physicians, and allowing for physicians' licenses to be suspended automatically in some cases (Schmidt 1988).

There is certainly a great deal of potential for further actions to identify and discipline incompetent medical care professionals. Such actions could take the pressure off insurance companies providing liability coverage for malpractice settlements, which would in turn minimize the adverse effects on access and cost escalation. Most importantly, disciplining professionals directly is more consistent with the intent of malpractice proceedings, providing an effective scheme of quality assurance.

Efforts to Improve Quality through Research

Scholars involved in health services research are able to make important contributions to discussions of what is necessary to assure the best possible quality of care for all patients. The potential contributions of research not based in clinical experimentation (which would be used when determining the efficacy of a new procedure) became apparent in the 1980s, thanks to the pioneering work of John Wennberg and others who reported the results of small area variations in the rates of certain medical procedures. For example, one study demonstrated wide variation in rates of hospitalization among children with asthma, toxic ingestions, and head injuries in Boston versus New Haven (Perrin et al. 1989). Although that particular study could not draw implications about the quality of care being offered in the various cities, the findings demonstrated the need for investigation of reasons for differences to see if one group was either under- or over-using hospital services.

Variations in some services raise even more concern about the quality of care, particularly if invasive procedures seem overused. Such is the case with variations in the rates of cesarean sections as the means of delivering babies. One study found that the rates of cesarean sections were the highest among non-Hispanic whites and lowest among Mexican Americans, and that the differences were statistically significant (Gould, Davy, and Stafford 1989). An extensive study of hospitalizations in thirteen sites found considerable variations in hospitalization rates for a variety of conditions, including total knee replacement, coronary-artery bypass surgery, destruction of benign skin lesions, and humeral fracture repair. The study controlled for the number of Medicare recipients in each area (the ratio was procedures per 10,000 Medicare patients). The authors concluded that the differences uncovered could not be explained by the data collected for their study, and that "correct" rates for the procedures investigated could not be established on the basis of existing data (Chassin et al. 1986). In research within a single state, Wennberg (1986) reported a 100 percent variation in rates of major cardiovascular surgery even though the incidence of ischemic heart disease was similar.

The implications of variations research are twofold. First, the differences in rates of procedures can easily be equated to differences in health care expenditures. Wennberg's study in Iowa found an average Medicare outlay of $1,002 in Iowa City and $1,753 in Des Moines (Wennberg 1986). Second, variations indicate a potential to reduce services in one area. In the case of cesarean sections, the consensus is that the rates are too high, disproportionately so in some communities. Data collected through variation studies can identify certain communities and/or institutions with particular potential for reducing their rates of procedures. For example, a hospital in Chicago implemented a requirement that there should be a second opinion before a cesarean section was performed, using objective criteria for four indications of cesarean section, and has begun detailed reviews of all operations and the physicians performing them. The program was successful in reducing the rate of cesarean sections from 17.5 percent to 11.5 percent (Myers and Gleicher 1988).

Aggregate data reveal differences in rates of using certain procedures to treat certain conditions; the obvious question becomes Which rate is appropriate? Answering that question requires analysis of individual case data, with the assistance of expert panels of clinical professionals to determine which procedure is most effective assuming certain conditions. Once that information is obtained, the research loop is completed. Given the new social and political environment, in which nonclinicians are more likely to question the judgment of physicians, there has been increased interest in involving public policymakers and health services researchers in the process of determining appropriate clinical guidelines for physicians. The research to determine those guidelines is conducted with the full participation of physicians and other health care providers, but implementing guidelines will be a process motivated by the public objectives of containing health care expenditures and assuring quality of care. The effort to improve the quality of medical care delivery through public investment in further research began in the mid- to late 1980s, with a special effort within the research grants and internal research programs of the Health Care Financing Administration. That agency, which manages the Medicare program in the federal government, has been working to develop measures of quality that are based on the outcomes from medical procedures and the use of medical care institutions. The objective of the effort is to be able to link the data collected in the Medicare program to measures of quality of care. Ultimately, this strategy will help consumers select health care providers and will help insurers, including the Medicare program, be confident of the return on their investments (Roper and Hackbarth 1988).

In 1989, the federal government embarked on a major effort to sponsor research designed to establish guidelines for medical practice. In the Omnibus Budget Reconciliation Act of 1989, Congress created a new agency, the Agency for Health Care Policy and Research (AHCPR), and mandated it to conduct and support research with respect to "the outcomes, effectiveness, and appropriateness of health care services and procedures" (House of Representatives 1989). The AHCPR has begun that effort, primarily by establishing and funding patient outcomes research teams (PORTs) focused on particular medical conditions. The PORTs are a part of a broader effort, the medical treatment effectiveness program (MEDTEP), which "consists of four elements: medical treatment effectiveness research, development of data bases for such research, development of clinical guidelines, and the dissemination of research findings and clinical guidelines" (Salive, Mayfield, and Weissman 1990). The initial work undertaken by PORTs will establish variations in rates of certain procedures. With that knowledge, the PORTs will conduct the research necessary to explain the reasons for the variations, which will ultimately contribute to defining the most appropriate rates. Seven PORTs have begun their work, studying procedures associated with the following conditions: acute myocardial infarction, benign prostatic hyperplasia and locally invasive prostatic carcinoma, lower back pain, cataracts, total knee replacement, chronic ischemic heart disease, and biliary tract disease (Salive, Mayfield, and Weissman 1990).

In addition to the activity of the PORTs, special panels of experts have been established to review the medical and health services literature specific to certain conditions, with the objective of developing practice guidelines. For example, a guideline panel has been formed to review the literature concerning the treatment of lower back pain. When their work is completed that panel will recommend certain guidelines for physicians to follow in treating this condition.

Research is under way, supported by the substantial commitment of public resources from Congress, to define medical practice guidelines and disseminate those guidelines to physicians. We can expect future reimbursement decisions to be made on the basis of those guidelines. The influence of physicians in developing public policy has both waned and shifted in recent years. The influence has waned as that of others in the issue network, particularly those concerned with cost containment, has increased. Research findings from small area studies have also accounted for a demystification of the practice of medicine, which has enabled laypersons to challenge intelligently the previously exclusive turf of physicians. The influence of physicians has shifted in that many of them now agree that clinical guidelines can be established and that they would be useful to health care professionals. Physicians are active participants in the PORTS. Being able to define quality standards by using the results of health services research is an idea whose time has come, after nearly twenty years of small area analysis. When Congress was searching for a means to address concerns about wide variations in health care outlays, a strategy was available and adopted by them.

Access to Quality Care and Organ Transplantation

Using research findings to develop clinical guidelines is a demonstration of the linkage between quality-of-care issues and cost containment. The case of organ transplantation is an illustration of the linkage between quality-of-care issues and access to health care services. There is some evidence that organ transplantation is a cost-effective alternative to other forms of treatment (Evans 1986), but the principal motivation for public policy has been to expand access to a procedure that without question improves the quality of life of many patients.[1]

Congressional interest in chronic organ failure began with the decision in 1972 to include kidney dialysis as a reimbursable expense in the Medicare program. That decision was followed by a policy to reimburse for the costs of kidney transplants, since that became a preferred means to treat the same condition. During the early 1980s, the use of transplantation as the preferred means of treating organ failure included organs other than kidneys, but federal payment policies lagged behind medical convention. Under policy directives, administrators of the Medicare program determine whether or not to include new medical procedures as reimbursable services after receiving advice from the Institute of Medicine, which conducts consensus conferences and reports results with recommendations to the Health Care Financing Administration. The latter agency was reluctant to include organ transplants as reimbursable services, admitting that cost considerations were included in their deliberations (Kosterlitz 1986).

By 1984, the demand for government action to assist those needing organ transplants was quite strong. The issue followed two paths to the institutional agenda in the federal government. First, direct appeals to the president for assistance in matching those needing transplants with potential donors were suc-

1. It should be noted that this reasoning does not yet apply to all transplants but instead to those that have proved clinical, not experimental, value in the judgment of the Institute of Medicine.

cessful and generated a great deal of public attention. Second, a policy entrepreneur, then-Representative Albert Gore, as chair of the Subcommittee on Investigation and Oversight of the Committee on Science and Technology, held hearings to both publicize the issue and develop policy options. He was assisted in this effort by a member of his staff who was a Robert Wood Johnson Foundation health policy fellow. This case, then, illustrates how an expanded issue network, combined with the ambitions of a policy entrepreneur, served to instigate policy action (Mueller 1989).

THE SPECIFICS OF POLICY DEVELOPMENT

The case of organ transplantation illustrates several important points made in this book about the development of public policy, and health policy more specifically. The manner in which the issue reached the institutional agenda, as already described, shows the roles of new actors in the issue network. Once it was on the agenda, other specialists in the issue network were influential in suggesting and developing particular components of the policy. Testimony by surgical experts convinced members of Congress that organ transplantation, at least in the cases of liver, heart, and heart-lung transplants, was no longer an experimental procedure.

The experts testifying before Representative Gore's subcommittee identified the most critical problem preventing increased access to transplants as matching a supply of organs to the demand for them. The problem had two facets. First, the total supply was inadequate to meet the demand. Second, the system of linking need and available organs was chaotic, without a single, nationwide means of locating available organs and delivering them to the location of the person in need. There were three regional organ procurement agencies in 1983, but they were not linked through any national network.

Issues of paying for transplants and the medication needed to prevent the rejection of new organs were also raised during legislative deliberations, but these concerns were outweighed by concerns about the availability of organs. The Medicare program was already paying for kidney transplants, and decisions on other organs were imminent. The most controversial funding decision related to payment for cyclosporine, the medication that helps prevent organ rejection.[2] That controversy continued until a legislative directive in 1986 to pay for the drug (Kosterlitz 1986).

2. A major difficulty in organ transplantation had been that the recipient's body would not recognize the new organ and would reject it with antibodies, causing infection and death. New medications have overcome that problem.

The progression of this legislation, from original draft to final passage as the Organ Transplantation Act of 1984, provides evidence of the importance of legislative compromises within the issue network that may be generally supportive of new initiatives. The original legislative suggestion included provisions restricting transplants to a small number of transplant centers and paying for cyclosporine, both of which were removed before final passage. The act was also not funded to the level of support desired by its supporters. Enough was in the legislation, however, to conclude that initial steps had been taken to establish national policy in a new area (Mueller 1989) and that a policy was established that deviated from other, procompetition measures taken during the 1980s (Blumstein 1989).

Actions taken since 1984 demonstrate the importance of policy implementation and considering policy design to be a never-ending process. The measures taken by Congress also illustrate how persistent policy entrepreneurs and others in an issue network can achieve their objectives through omnibus legislation once an original enabling act is passed that can be amended. One such amendment was enacted in 1986 as part of the Omnibus Budget Reconciliation Act of that year. This amendment compelled hospitals to provide notification to family members of the opportunity to donate organs of dying kin (Blumstein 1989). The same act included a provision to pay for immunosuppressive drugs following a transplant. In the 1988 reauthorization of this program, a final piece of the original mosaic was included, a bone-marrow registry (Mueller 1989).

PROBLEMS IN POLICY IMPLEMENTATION

The 1984 legislation supported a national network of organ procurement agencies (OPAS), to be coordinated by the private United Network for Organ Sharing (UNOS). The purpose of this scheme was to guarantee coordination of effort when an individual was in need of a particular organ, regardless of where the individual was or where the available organ might be. All health care providers wishing to receive public reimbursement for organ transplants and/or providing organs for transplants must be members of this organization. The criteria for membership are determined by UNOS, not a duly constituted agency of the federal government. Some have argued that this concession of what amounts to government regulatory power to a nongovernment entity is an inappropriate use of government authority and that the result may even constitute a violation of antitrust policies (Blumstein 1989). Organizational battles between the private UNOS and the public agency administering Medicare, HCFA, have been protracted but may ease with the passage of time and the reaching of new agreements (Mueller 1989).

Implementation of the 1984 legislation was also plagued by budget debates forcing limits in available dollars and by interbranch disagreements between Congress and the Reagan administration between 1984 and 1987. Members of Congress, as evident in their remarks during committee hearings in 1986 and 1987, were more than a little dismayed with administrative delays in implementing the program to provide grants to OPAs and in setting up a national network for sharing available organs. In the opinion of some members, including Senator Kennedy, administrative inaction was inexcusable, given clear and specific statements of congressional intent in the original legislation. This point was particularly applicable to the delays in establishing the grant program for OPAs (Mueller 1989).

SUMMARY: LESSONS FOR LEGISLATIVE INVOLVEMENT IN ACCESS TO HIGH TECHNOLOGY

In 1984 Congress took action in an effort to facilitate use of a technology-intensive medical procedure, organ transplantation. The intent was to assure access to high-quality medical care, symbolized by the technology of which American medicine is rightly proud. Did Congress succeed? Are there implications for future actions of this type?

Congress succeeded, after an interval of time to overcome organizational problems, in establishing a national network for sharing organs. The objective of dramatically increasing the supply of organs available for donations, however, was not met. A report in 1988 detailed the following unmet demand for organs: 4,000 corneas, 600 hearts, 430 livers, and 140 heart/lungs (Fackelmann 1988). Public policy may not be an appropriate means of encouraging the very private act of donating organs; of the 22,000 annual brain deaths, only 4,000 result in organ donations (Fackelmann 1988).

The implications for future action are twofold. First, Congress has learned to use the expanded issue network to play a more direct role in writing the details of programs to specify public interventions in complex processes. The fact that organ transplantations represent sophisticated medicine, and that setting up a national network requires complex administrative decision making, have not inhibited members of Congress from enacting public policies. In the development of national organ transplant policy we have seen how the expansion of congressional staffing has affected the ability of members of Congress to challenge directly what they perceive to be foot dragging by members of the administration.

We have also seen Congress quite concerned about the availability of high-technology procedures for all citizens. In order to accommodate the legislative process, normally slow and deliberate, with technological advances, which can be quite rapid, Congress used the vehicles of omnibus legislation and extensive oversight of administrative agencies. Passing legislation while the opportunity is present and then modifying it with subsequent amendments are a means of overcoming the problems Diebold (1984) saw in how our social institutions attempt to keep pace with changes in biomedicine.

Finally, the case of organ transplantation illustrates the desire of public officials to make proven medical procedures widely available and not tolerate rationing of those procedures. Without policy intervention, organ transplants are effectively rationed to those able to secure organs and those able to finance the immunosuppressive medications needed following the procedure. Efforts such as the Organ Transplantation Act of 1984 and subsequent amendments may evade debates about rationing procedures and diverting resources to other uses, but they do demonstrate the commitment to supporting the initiatives in biomedicine to improve quality of care.

Prevention as the Means to High-Quality Health

Preventing ill health is preferable to treating conditions that could have been prevented. These three types of activities should be included in a comprehensive effort to prevent ill health: promoting good health through appropriate behavior, eliminating or at least reducing environmental hazards that contribute to ill health, and controlling chronic health problems to prevent crisis conditions.

HEALTH PROMOTION

Policies designed to increase activities that promote good health are targeted to individual behavior. Smoking cessation programs are designed to eliminate a specific behavior known to be related to the onset of several critical illnesses, including cancer, heart problems, and chronic obstructive lung disease (COLD). Data published by the U.S. Office of Disease Prevention and Health Promotion demonstrate that smoking has the following consequences:

- accounts for 30 percent of all cancer deaths
- accounts for 25 percent of all cancer deaths in women
- is the major cause of COLD in the United States

• is the major cause of coronary heart disease in the United States
• increases the risk for cardiac death two- to fourfold
• costs between $38 and $95 billion annually in health expenditures and lost productivity (Office of Disease Prevention and Health Promotion 1988).
The benefits of smoking cessation are obvious, given those facts. For those who discontinue smoking, rates of coronary heart disease and general mortality rates decline to levels similar to those of nonsmokers (Office of Disease Prevention and Health Promotion 1988).

Smoking cessation represents activities designed to discontinue bad health behavior; ending alcohol and drug abuse are other examples. Other promotion activities emphasize adopting new behaviors. A good example is to increase exercise activities. Exercise can improve health by controlling body weight, improving cardiovascular health, increasing bone density (preventing osteoporosis), reducing blood glucose levels, and reducing the likelihood of depression (Office of Disease Prevention and Health Promotion 1988).

Individuals can achieve good health and avoid adverse conditions through behavior related to health promotion. Physical exercise and other promotion activities can help individuals attain and maintain optimum weight, blood pressure, blood cholesterol levels, and mental health (Breslow 1990).

ELIMINATING OR REDUCING ENVIRONMENTAL HAZARDS

Significant advances have been made throughout history by eliminating agents in the environment known to cause poor health. A good example is controlling the presence of raw sewage in public places, and another is cleaning water before making it available for consumption. Much work remains, however. The U.S. Environmental Protection Agency continues to monitor the quality of the air and water and reports cities and states that are not in compliance with federal standards. During 1983 the level of ozone exceeded standards an average of 11.4 days in sites across the United States, and carbon monoxide levels exceeded the standard an average of 7.7 days (Office of Disease Prevention and Health Promotion 1988). Reports of contamination of the nation's water continue, with the following pollutants most typically reported: bacteria, biochemical oxygen demand, nutrients, total suspended solids, toxics, metals, acidity, salinity, and ammonia (Office of Disease Prevention and Health Promotion 1988). These data represent public health problems that require, at a minimum, continuous monitoring. If any environmental conditions precipitate a large health crisis, new policies may be needed.

An area of concern related to environmental factors is that of occupational health. Certain industries experience higher rates of accidents than others, particularly agriculture and construction. Strategies to prevent ill health should include policies to reduce the risk associated with occupational activities. Similarly, reducing rates of motor vehicle accidents should also be considered to be an activity of public health related to prevention.

CONTROLLING CHRONIC HEALTH PROBLEMS

Certain medical services extend good health by controlling chronic health problems. This is a strategy designed to prevent acute episodes of illness such as heart attacks or strokes among those persons with chronic high blood pressure. The health care system can take preventative action by doing the following:

• including routine checks for signs of chronic conditions, such as measuring blood pressure and cholesterol levels

• providing immunization services to children

• providing counseling services to prospective mothers regarding prenatal care

There are two direct policy implications in considering strategies to promote regular check-ups for early signs of chronic conditions and routine care when such conditions develop. First, public health agencies should make some services available through clinics free to the public. This is especially true of immunization and routine checks of blood pressure. Second, public policymakers should continue to support preventive services through publically financed programs such as Medicare and Medicaid. Further, public policymakers should consider requiring that such services be included in all basic insurance policies offered through employers and other sources.

SUMMARY

At a time when much of the policy debate surrounding health care issues is driven by the ever-increasing expenditures for medical services, we should pay special attention to policies promoting good health. For example, one recently published study estimated that adults aged twenty-five and over incur $2,342 per smoker in health expenditures they would not otherwise have experienced. This aggregates to $187 billion in five years in excess expenditures related to smoking (Hodgson 1992). A cost reduction policy, then, should be to promote good health behavior.

Promoting good health will also improve the quality of life of individuals, which is the ultimate objective of public health policy. By promoting good health we can also reduce the incidence of ill health spreading from one person to another. This is certainly the case in preventing communicable diseases through immunization. Finally, public policies designed to provide opportunities to change behavior and/or receive preventive services are expanding access to health care services. The three goals of health policy—cost containment, quality, and access—can all be well served by policies related to preventing ill health. Those policies will not achieve one goal at the expense of others.

Conclusion

There has always been an interest among policymakers to assure citizens that a minimum quality of care standards will be enforced in the patient-provider interaction. During the 1970s and into the 1980s, however, the concern about escalating health expenditures dominated policy debates. By the end of the 1980s, the debates had expanded to include access to health care as an issue, particularly for the uninsured, the elderly, and residents of rural communities. As the 1990s have begun, a discussion of quality of care has been added to this policy mixture, especially in the context of the malpractice crisis, medical effectiveness research, use of advanced technologies in health care, and consequences of earlier efforts to control health care expenditures.

This overview of issues concerning quality has included instances in which the general arguments made early in this book about the development of public policies could be applied to particular policies. The discussion of malpractice is an example of establishing national policy through the police powers of the separate states. The discussion of medical effectiveness research demonstrates how Congress is able to undertake major new initiatives in the context of budget-driven public policies. By amending the Omnibus Budget Reconciliation Act, Congress is able to create substantive direction for how dollars are spent, in this case to create new funds and direct them to research on medical effectiveness. The interest in this research is an illustration of matching legislative interest in a subject with an idea the research community has generated and integrated into discussions, an idea whose time has come. Small area research has demonstrated the value of identifying the variations in medical practice, and that approach is now the building block of medical effectiveness research.

The issue of public support for organ transplantation, including increasing the supply of organs and helping to finance the procedures, is an appropriate lens through which to see most clearly the final point of this chapter, the blending of quality, access, and cost-containment emphases in current and future health policy. Quality-of-care concerns are most immediate in determining whether or not the new procedures are appropriate treatments (for the federal government this involves determining whether or not they are experimental). The issue of quality blends with access to care when the policy objectives are to assure the highest quality treatment is available to all who need it. This concern led directly to the passage of the Organ Transplantation Act of 1984. Concerns about cost containment enter the discussion when the government considers paying for part or all of the service, as it did with immunosuppressive drugs in 1986 (Mueller 1989).

There may be times when the emphasis on delivering the highest quality of care possible may clash with concerns about cost containment and/or access to care. The latter will be true when society lacks the resources, such as a supply of organs, needed to make new procedures widely available. The high costs of procedures taking advantage of the latest technological advances in care raise the specter of cost containment when decisions are made to declare the procedures nonexperimental, making them eligible for Medicare reimbursement. It has become impossible to enact policies advancing one of the three major objectives—quality, access, or cost containment—without considering the implications for achieving the other two.

Policies accounting for the trade-offs among objectives will be efforts to make decisions concerning the total benefits to society of one course of action over another. This approach takes the decisions out of the context of interactions between individual providers and patients, and even out of the context of sets of providers (such as hospitals or nursing homes) and consumers. Jonsen (1990) has made a persuasive argument that a "new medicine" exists that departs from our traditional notions of one-on-one interactions between a doctor and his/her patient. Instead, medical decisions are now based on determining procedures that treat classes of patients.

Policymakers should also change the way they approach their tasks, based on the same changes in medicine and changes in what society can afford to tolerate in public expenditures. The first step is to recognize the implications of narrow decisions on the more general nature of health care delivery. This would mean, for example, not enacting a new payment for one sector of the health care delivery system until the implications of that change for others in the system are explored. The second step is to consider just what society should finance through publicly funded programs. Policymakers in the state of Oregon are engaged in just such a discussion vis-à-vis that state's Medicaid program (Southwick 1990). Legislators in Colorado are considering a similar measure (McEachern 1990). As a nation, we are not yet explicitly debating rationing of health care. Our decisions as to whether or not specific new services will be considered benefits of programs such as Medicare, however, are implicit rationing decisions.

The balance of quality, access, and cost containment is becoming more difficult to maintain now that all three are simultaneously high-priority public objectives. This chapter has described some of the leading issues in establishing and maintaining the highest possible quality in the delivery of medical care. Although some changes designed to improve quality, such as more effective programs to discipline physicians and medical effectiveness guidelines, might save public dollars (because of fewer malpractice suits and less unnecessary surgery), other efforts to provide quality care, such as organ transplants, add costs. At some point in time, we may well need to establish a minimum standard of quality that we would like made available to all citizens.

7

. . .

Health Care Reform:
Lessons from Abroad
and National Health Insurance

Previous chapters have described U.S. health policies as they currently exist. The overall picture is a mosaic of specific policies enacted to address particular problems in the interactions between health care providers and consumers of their services. Although there have been general themes in health care policy— monitoring quality of care, assuring access to care, and containing health care costs—there has not been a unified national policy. As a nation we have at various times asked but never answered the question: What ought to be the national policy in health care? As one of only two industrialized nations without national health insurance (South Africa is the other), the United States has implicitly supported a fragmented system of delivering and financing health care. As we approach the twenty-first century, numerous interest groups and members of Congress are promoting new policies to change health care financing and organization.

Many of the suggested reforms are modeled on experiences in other nations, particularly in those that offer comprehensive services without the U.S. experience of dramatic increases in expenditures. The systems used in Western European nations and Canada are of particular interest, with the latter receiving the most attention in recent years. In this chapter, I will provide an overview of those systems and describe proposals being debated in the United States.

Health Policies in Other Nations
During the 1960s and into the 1970s, U.S. policymakers and others promoting national health insurance were excited about the possibilities of learning from the experiences of Great Britain. Research findings, however, revealed a prac-

tice of rationing care, for example kidney transplants were not available to persons aged fifty-five or older (Aaron and Schwartz 1984). The British solution to the problem of financing health care was dismissed because not all care was publicly financed. Policymakers in the United States can benefit from the British experience as well as other plans that offer comprehensive benefits through a variety of schemes. The Canadian system achieves favorable health statistics (such as life expectancy, infant mortality, and other general population measures) while spending far less money per person than the U.S. health care system. Elements of the Canadian system may be transferrable to the United States.

WESTERN EUROPEAN SYSTEMS

Comparisons of per capita health expenditures among industrialized nations consistently show those in the United States to be the highest. After controlling for differences in currency values, in 1987, the U.S. per capita cost of health care was $2,051, compared to $1,090 in France, $1,073 in Germany, $884 in Italy, and $746 in the United Kingdom (Schieber 1990). At the same time, the health care systems in other nations at least implicitly guarantee access to health care for all citizens. This match of lower costs and universal access is quite appealing to American policymakers and analysts interested in resolving the problems plaguing the system in this nation. The United States could certainly benefit from the experiences of other nations in controlling aggregate health care expenditures. Lest we become too excited about the benefits of nationalized systems, we must also recognize the costs, potential and real, of adopting a system organized and managed by the government.

Universal access in nationalized systems leads to increased use, which in turn affects health outcomes in those nations. In Sweden, for example, all mothers can visit a free child health clinic for the first two years after giving birth. In the French system, mothers receive prenatal and postnatal family allowance grants and paid maternity leave of between ten and twenty-eight weeks. Both financial benefits can help mothers with the time and expense associated with appropriate medical care. These policies help explain lower infant mortality rates in other Western nations compared to the results achieved in the United States. Although access is unquestionably universal for most services in other nations, there are still differences in access across income groups and working environments (Adrian 1985; Wysong and Abel 1990).

The most important difference across countries is between those that pay for health care through private sources and those that pay through public sources. A government payment system creates a scheme whereby a single source controls all revenue funneled to health care professionals, which is a means for creating a direct assault on the bills for services rendered by those providers. Providers can request all the money they desire, but they will have to accept the payment given by the single payer. This scheme has been judged by some to be more effective than the procompetition approach taken by the U.S. government in the 1980s (Pfaff 1990). A single payer will exercise monopsony power to control expenditures. There will be inevitable exceptions to the rule that all provider income will be derived from that payer, but the additional payments, either through a black market or through outside payment permitted by the national system, will be minimal.

Specific lessons in financing health care can be gleaned from the experiences of other nations. The United States, as discussed in Chapter 3, is moving toward a scheme of paying for physicians' services based on the relative value of those services, regardless of the specialization of the physician. The values will be based on the resource consumption needed to provide specific services. Germany (formerly West Germany) has been using a similar system since 1978. The German plan includes determinations of the values of specific services, negotiations between the government and physicians, and the use of an expenditure cap to control overall spending for physicians' services. An overall level of expenditures for physicians' services is set by the government, after negotiations with physicians. This cap serves to control both the charges for services and the total volume of services rendered. Physicians' groups negotiate rates and total amounts with government officials and are then left to influence their own colleagues to live within the predetermined levels of reimbursement (Kirkman-Liff 1990).

Important cultural and political differences help explain the success of nationalized systems in other countries and the lack of similar initiatives in the United States Those same differences should make us rather cautious about the prospects of adopting directly the approaches of other nations. In Germany, for example: "The change in policy to limit expenditures on physician reimbursement and to segment fee-for-service pools to discourage excessive laboratory testing signifies a decline in the political power of physicians vis-à-vis other corporate interests" (Kirkman-Liff 1990, 91). The political culture in the United States, which is characterized by interest groups seeking to maximize their own gains in a competitive political arena, contrasts starkly with other nations such as the United Kingdom, which can be characterized as bargaining arenas in which groups expect to negotiate with others (Eckstein 1960).

Important differences in the preferences of physicians in the various nations help explain the ability of the American Medical Association to resist national health insurance whereas in other nations, physicians have been partners in nationalized systems. In Great Britain, for example, the principal concern of physicians has been the ability to practice with complete freedom from any interference from professional colleagues. They are willing to work with the government in exchange for government protection from pressures to form medical practice groups or follow practice guidelines developed by other physicians (Lister 1986; Eckstein 1960).

Important differences exist across Western nations in how government decisions are made and the expectations for government influence in social policies such as health care. Many Western nations operate within a democratic corporatist model of decision making, wherein government, business, and labor merge to form a social partnership. In that framework, government officials, and civil servants in particular, can play a dominant role in policymaking. This is the approach to decision making in Germany and Sweden. Other nations, such as France, adopt an even more proactive role for government as the central planner for social policy. In this model, government decides the general interests of all of society and develops policies accordingly. Finally, other nations follow a market model in which civil servants do not play a major role in the policy process and in which groups are in conflict and operate with autonomy from government control. In those systems, though, the relative power of groups may vary such that in some societies (Great Britain and Canada, in particular) the interests of business groups may dominate (Adrian 1985). Decision making in corporatist and planning cultures will often lead to major policy enactments such as national health insurance. In two of the nations Adrian identified as market model societies, Canada and Great Britain, there are elements of corporatist mentality that have influenced the development of national health policies.

In the British and Canadian systems, as well as in other Western nations, the parliamentary system of government has facilitated consideration of more holistic policies than the normal U.S. consideration of incremental change. In the American system, a general distrust of political solutions to problems has helped restrict government activities to "a bit of tinkering and some new incentives" (Morone 1990b, 133). Even when fairly drastic policy measures are taken, such as changing the means of reimbursing hospitals, those measures are not approached as direct political choices. Instead, they are treated as administrative adjustments in the existing system (Morone 1990b).

THE CANADIAN SYSTEM

There may be greater opportunity to learn from the experiences of Canada than from those of other Western nations, because Canada is more similar to the United States socially and politically. Canada, like the United States, is a federal system, with provinces playing roles similar to those of the states. Canada is also heterogenous, although not as much so as the United States. Canada is geographically large and experiences similar problems to the United States in delivering services to remote rural areas.

The Canadian system of national health insurance experiences lower expenditures per capita than does the U.S. system, and spends a smaller percentage of its gross domestic product on health care—8.6 percent versus 11.2 percent in the United States in 1987 (Evans 1990). This difference began in 1971, when Canadian provinces established single-payer systems; before that year expenditures between the two nations were quite similar. Canadian citizens enjoy universal access to essential health care services—at least that is the impression. Since this system is touted as a model for action in the United States, it warrants special attention in this discussion of what the U.S. policy ought to be.

The development of the Canadian system, particularly the involvement of government policy directly in financial arrangements with physicians and other health professionals, can be traced back to the 1930s. The government made payments directly to physicians to compensate for any unpaid medical bills. During the 1930s, general practitioners worked on salary as municipal employees in sixty-seven locations in Saskatchewan, five in Manitoba, and three in Alberta. Rather than designing systems similar to Medicaid wherein the state pays providers for each service to eligible clients, in the 1930s, Canadian provinces initiated systems that paid physicians a flat fee each month for each eligible person in their practice. The Canadian Medical Association cooperated fully in developing schemes of government insurance. By the end of the 1940s, precedents had been set that favored government-sponsored insurance, cooperation between government and the medical profession in planning government insurance programs, and public support of government-financed insurance plans (80 percent of those polled in 1944 stated they would contribute to a national hospital-medical insurance plan) (Taylor 1978). These precedents differ from those set in the United States with the early development of private health care insurance and the later addition of government programs that pay on the basis of each specific service delivered.

The development of national health insurance in Canada was not a smooth road from the early initiatives in the 1930s to a national system in the 1970s. The medical profession opposed further government action during the 1950s and 1960s, going so far as to close physicians' offices in Saskatchewan in 1962 (Naylor 1986). The national system in Canada followed actions by separate provinces, beginning with a hospital insurance program in Saskatchewan in 1946 that paved the way for a national hospital program in 1961 and national medical plan in 1971. The national system is an amalgamation of separate provincial plans that receive federal financial support, similar to the U.S. scheme with Medicaid. The critical difference is that in Canada all citizens are included in the government plan, versus only the very poor in the U.S. Medicaid program.

Saskatchewan also pioneered the addition of medical insurance to the basic plan and was the first province to control directly the fees paid to doctors. While the traditional fee-for-service system was retained for the purposes of calculating payment, fees were tightly controlled by the government. The scheme of bargaining between the provincial government and representatives of various groups of medical professionals (such as general practice physicians, surgeons, allied health professionals) began with the Saskatchewan plan and remains in place today. The Canadian system took many years to develop:

> One cannot fail to be impressed by the length of time it took for the desire to be transformed into operating programs. As long ago as 1919, the idea had received sufficient support to become a stated plank in the Liberal party platform. But it was to take another half-century—almost two generations—for health insurance to become a nation-wide reality. (Taylor 1978, 421)

Supporters of national health insurance in the United States can take heart in how long it took the Canadian system to develop; perhaps we are on the same time line in this country.

There are important differences, though, in the development of health care policy in the two nations. Foremost among them has been the activity of the professional associations, particularly the American Medical Association and the Canadian Medical Association. The latter is much more inclined to accept at least some government involvement in payment for medical bills and has designed its lobbying strategies to accommodate rather than oppose government decision making (Naylor 1986). The two nations are also different in their cultural acceptance of government influence in decisions affecting the delivery of medical care (Kosterlitz 1989a). There are other obvious differences, particularly in population; the total population in Canada is slightly more than 10 percent of the U.S. population. Designing comprehensive systems may be easier when smaller populations are served. There are also differences in the nature of the health care delivery and financing system. The U.S. system has evolved into a much more fragmented collage of different providers, both institutions and individual professionals. When the Canadian system was developed, there were very few separate parties involved in paying for health care; private insurance plans existed but were few in number and did not cover as a high a percentage of the total population as is the case in the United States today. During the 1950s and 1960s, the technological explosion had not yet reached health care and designing a system of payment was simpler than it is today. In short, policymakers in the United States face a much different political, social, and economic environment than did Canadian officials in the 1960s.

It may not be practical to consider adopting the Canadian plan wholesale for financing health care in the United States, but important lessons can nevertheless be drawn from the Canadian experience. The most important is that medical care expenditures can be controlled. There are several reasons expenditures are less in Canada and some of them could be transferred to the U.S. system. First, there is less administrative expense in the Canadian system because there are no overhead costs from multiple insurers as there are in the United States, and there is less paperwork required for reimbursement since fees are set in advance. Second, physician fees are tightly controlled in Canada, through negotiations between physicians' groups and provincial government officials. Third, hospital use and technology are controlled in Canada and therefore limited (Evans, 1990). The success of the Canadian controls can be seen in the divergence of price increases between Canada and the United States since 1971. In that year, health spending in Canada was 7.4 percent of gross domestic product and in the United States, 7.6 percent. By 1981 the same figures were 7.7 percent and 9.2 percent, and in 1987, 8.6 percent and 11 percent (Evans et al. 1989). Examining one component of the health care delivery system, per-capita spending for hospital care in the United States in 1985 was $680, compared to $460 in Canada (Newhouse, Anderson, and Roos 1988).

Can we achieve some of Canada's success? The new scheme for reimbursing physicians in the Medicare program borrows some concepts from Canada. The initial fees are determined differently, relying on a "technical fix" through the resource-based relative-value scale. Considerations are being given to include either volume controls or expenditure ceilings, both ideas that are being used in Canadian provinces. Cultural differences explain the different strategies used by the two governments. In the Canadian system, where the government is closer to the corporatist model described by Adrian and where the medical profession has a history of working with government officials, bargaining is used. In the United States, where government involvement is more difficult to justify, there is a greater effort to set fees according to some objective, scientific criteria. Although the U.S. government can replicate some of the Canadian experience in controlling physicians' payments, overall health care expenditures may not be affected. Just as the effective Medicare controls on hospital payments have only shifted payment to other sources, either to other payers or to other sites for patient care, Medicare restrictions on physicians' payment may result in costs shifting to insurers and the use of health professionals other than physicians, those whose prices are not yet controlled. The complexity of the delivery system once again works against efforts to control costs, and the perceived Canadian panacea may not be replicable in the United States.

The perception of Canadian success in cost containment masks problems that should serve as warning signals to U.S. policymakers as more drastic health policy reforms are considered in this nation. Hospital expenditures are less in Canada than in the United States, in large part because the quantity of hospital services is rationed in the former nation. Universal coverage is provided in Canada, meaning all citizens, regardless of income, are entitled to the same services. Those services, however, are rationed according to the perceived need for particular treatments. There are far fewer hospital beds per one thousand people in Canada than in the United States, which has meant that the beds occupied by patients requiring chronic care are not available for others; occupancy in Ontario hospitals is 94 percent, compared with 60 percent in U.S. hospitals (Kosterlitz 1989b). Expensive equipment—such as magnetic resonance imaging equipment and lithotripters, which crush kidney stones—is limited in number. As a result of the limits on beds and equipment, patients must wait months for services, sometimes even years. Some hospital patients have had to lie on stretchers in hospital hallways and do without amenities such as hospital-provided pillows.

Nonemergency procedures are also delayed, sometimes several months in the case of cardiac surgery (Kosterlitz 1989b). Certain dramatic cases have been publicized that are the end results of the delays. In 1989, a patient died after finally undergoing bypass surgery that had been delayed since the beginning of 1988, and rescheduled eleven times. In the Toronto area in 1989, there were one thousand patients waiting for six to eight months for bypass surgery (Witt 1989). Some Canadian residents with particular problems are crossing the border into the United States for medical care, for example from Windsor into Detroit for bypass surgery; an agency in Windsor referred 147 patients to U.S. hospitals between May 1989 and February 1990 (*Detroit Free Press* 1990). In sum, universal access remains the objective of the Canadian system, but there are restrictions on the nature of the care available.

The Canadian strategy for controlling costs is attractive, particularly because it might successfully limit the rapid expansion of technology (Stark 1988). The principle weakness in that strategy is that the balances being struck might become restrictions on surgery and other uses of hospitals. A second weakness in the strategy is that by relying on government as the sole payer for health care services, funds devoted to health care become subject to the political and economic constraints affecting government spending. Even though health care expenditures have been controlled in Canada, they still outpaced inflation in eight years of the last thirteen (Iglehart 1990). The federal government has reduced its contributions to the provincial governments, putting a great deal of pressure on them. This may well become a critical problem in the future of the Canadian system:

> But it seems inevitable that Canada will eventually reopen the question of how care is financed. The provinces will jeopardize their capacity to support other social priorities if they continue to rely on tax revenues to finance unlimited access to most health services, and to produce more physicians than can be accommodated. (Iglehart 1990, 568)

The risk of financing the health program exclusively with government funds is that health care must then compete with other social programs and needs of the government, especially in times when the government must reduce its spending commitments. Despite cost-per-service controls and expenditure ceilings, increases in health care expenditures can exceed general economic growth, as has been the case in Canada. Since government revenues are a function of general economic growth, this reality can leave government coffers short when the time comes to pay the health care bills. Canadian provinces began to feel the crunch in 1991 and looked to the United States for specific means of controlling expenditures. In the largest province of Ontario, health care resources, including hospital beds, were reduced (*New York Times* 1991). Policy leaders there may need to adopt different payment schemes and begin asking specific questions about the costs of specific services, as is being done in the United States.

SUMMARY

Advocates of reforming the methods of delivering and financing health care in the United States will inevitably press for systems more closely resembling those of other Western nations. It is a common criticism of the United States that it is joined only by South Africa as industrialized nations without national health insurance. Suggestions to simply adopt the scheme of national health insurance used by another nation, however, generate a great deal of debate because there are generally flaws in the other systems that critics of national health insurance can use as ammunition in their arguments.

The trade-offs between stringent cost control and access to quality care are obvious after closer observation of nationalized systems. Perhaps nowhere is the trade-off more obvious now than in the Canadian system. Pressures to control health care expenditures have led to health care rationing based on need for services. Even after rationing, the costs of health care still pose serious financial problems for provincial governments. The Canadian system provides lessons in the problem of financing technological advances in medical treatment. In that system technology is rationed, which leads to waiting lists to receive services. Simply put, there is no inexpensive way to provide health care to a nation's population.

Although there is no panacea, other systems should be examined carefully for specific elements that could be adapted to the U.S. health care system. Different methods of paying for care could be adopted here, as is currently being done within the Medicare program for the reimbursement of physicians. Policymakers in the United States can also avoid pitfalls of other systems, especially service limitations that lead to adverse health care outcomes. As long as proponents of national health insurance carry the argument forward stated in terms that either we have or do not have a system similar to that of Canada or other nations, these more subtle means of benefiting from comparisons will be lost in the swirl of argument and controversy fueled by the examples of lower cost on the one hand and deaths from rationing on the other.

National Health Care Reform in the United States

For those who advocate reform of the health care delivery and finance systems in American health care, there is cause for optimism. The American public seems primed for change. A national survey in 1990 found that 29 percent of the American public favored completely rebuilding the health care system and 60 percent favored fundamental changes. As an indication of the specific changes envisioned by the public, 66 percent preferred the Canadian system to the U.S. system, which was an increase from the 61 percent who favored it two years earlier (Blendon et al. 1990). By 1992, health care reform became a viable political issue. The election of Senator Wofford in Pennsylvania in a special election in 1991 was a forerunner of the heated discussion of health care reform in the election season of 1992. The American public, according to one survey, saw health care as the number-two issue after concerns about the economy. A majority of respondents in that poll were concerned that health insurance would become too expensive to purchase and that expensive bills would not be covered by private insurance (Smith et al. 1992). During the presidential primaries of early 1992, health care reform was an important issue among Democrats, with Senator Bob Kerrey of Nebraska using it as the keystone issue in his campaign. The debate continued after the party conventions in the summer as the incumbent (Bush) advocated a market-based reform using tax incentives and the challenger (Clinton) advocated a government mandate that employers provide insurance.

HEALTH CARE REFORM PROPOSALS IN THE 1980S

The cumulative effects of recent policies are already leading this nation in the direction of substantive reform, both in terms of access to care through government-sponsored programs and in terms of how health care is financed. There were sharp criticisms of health policy in the early years of the Ronald Reagan presidency, and health programs seemed more likely to be cut than were other programs (Iglehart 1985). There was certainly reason to be pessimistic: in the Omnibus Budget Reconciliation Act of 1981 the Medicaid program was reduced by restricting eligibility, and in reconciliation acts since then, the Medicare program has absorbed spending reductions. These reductions, even though they are reductions from projected expenditures and not reductions from current-year amounts, have generated a great deal of controversy. The elderly in particular have objected to deficit reductions being passed on disproportionately to the Medicare program. With all the public attention given to the debates concerning budget cuts, we may easily lose sight of the positive steps taken in the 1980s to reform the system.

The most dramatic changes have occurred in health care financing. In 1983, Congress established the prospective payment system (PPS) to reimburse hospitals for care provided to Medicare patients. The Medicare program has been used to influence behavior by physicians and others who control the length of stay in hospitals and the resources used during those hospital stays. Although the overall program continues to experience dramatic cost increases because of continued increases in the use of a variety of medical services, the PPS must nevertheless be recognized as a major government initiative to reform health care financing. Earlier chapters in this book discussed some evidence of trade-offs between cost containment and quality of care that occurred in the early years of the PPS. In communities with few or no alternatives to hospitals as providers of extended care, early discharges from hospitals can be detrimental to the patient's health. Those problems, however, have been minimal.

In 1989 Congress enacted a reform, currently being phased in, to change the rules for reimbursing physicians under the Medicare program by adopting a resource-based relative value system to pay for services rendered by physicians. Once again a major change has occurred in health care financing as a result of government action. Both changes in Medicare reimbursement have far-reaching implications since they can be copied by others who pay for health care. Specifically, state governments often follow the lead of the Medicare program in setting reimbursement policies for the Medicaid program. Major insurance carriers also often adopt ideas first tested by the Medicare program. These changes are all incremental in the sense that they are not enacted as elements in a holistic change in policies concerning health care delivery and finance, but their cumulative effect can nonetheless be quite significant.

The measures designed to contain increases in health expenditures have been at least modestly effective. They are now being used as the building blocks of proposals that would expand access to medical care services and at the same time constrain expenditures. The Medicare cost-containment reforms have been efforts to determine equitable prices for services rendered by medical care providers. When combined with elements of volume controls, these policies provide the financial flexibility to consider dramatic expansions of access to services.

In addition to activities to change health care finance, the federal government was actively expanding public programs in the 1980s, despite the rhetoric of budget reductions and less government involvement in our lives. During the second half of that decade various federal laws included provisions that expanded the eligibility for Medicaid to include all children in families with incomes below 135 percent of poverty, provided federal funds for medications needed following organ transplants, expanded programs in child and maternal health, added new catastrophic benefits to the Medicare program, and compelled employers to offer insurance at group rates to employees and spouses of employees whose services are terminated. These activities have been labelled a "new activism" by Brown (1990), an interpretation that is entirely appropriate.

State governments have also been active in addressing issues of health care delivery and access. The most dramatic examples have been those states that adopted programs designed to move public policy closer to universal access. Of particular note have been policies enacted in Hawaii, Florida, and Massachusetts. Brown (1990) points to programs creating risk pools for high-risk persons and expansion in Medicaid eligibility as examples of new activism by state governments.

Why have we seen this activity, even in an era of an ideology favoring limited government? There are several explanations. The problems of health care access have become too obvious for government to ignore. Researchers have helped us realize the difficulties the uninsured have in obtaining access to health care, and the number of uninsured grew during the 1980s and continues to grow. Health care expenditures continue to grow rapidly, forcing major payers for health care—and the federal government is the largest single payer—to look for more and more radical means of controlling those expenditures. In short, there have been intense pressures to adopt more radical reforms of the system.

Resistance to those reforms has diminished somewhat in recent years because the lobbying strength of the medical professions has lessened in comparison to the voices of those who demand change. The comparative loss of power is the result of two factors. First, the profession has become more decentralized into different, smaller groups. When policies are debated that would favor one group of health professionals over another, as was the case with both major payment reforms of the 1980s, the medical profession has a much more difficult time lobbying against those suggestions. Second, the power of other groups has increased in proportion to the perceived seriousness of the problems being addressed. Thus, the power of insurance companies and state governments in arguing for cost controls increases as health care expenditure increases continue unabated. The influence of policy advocates arguing on behalf of the uninsured increases as the numbers of the uninsured increase.

The political environment changed dramatically during the 1980s. The proliferation in Congress of platforms from which to advance a policy gave more credence to the arguments of policy entrepreneurs such as then-Representative Albert Gore. The influence of these members of Congress, and of key subcommittee chairmen such as Henry Waxman and Pete Stark in the House of Representatives, grew when two successive Republican presidents chose not to involve themselves heavily in domestic policy. Those presidents were especially reluctant to suggest new alternatives, with the single exception of the Medicare Catastrophic Care Act. The annual use of budget reconciliation created an opportunity to offer specific changes to government programs that would not themselves be the subject of lengthy committee deliberations and possible blockage by interest groups with particular clout. Instead, reconciliation can be used as a vehicle to attach any "budget-neutral" item, which then becomes part of the total bill that is voted on as a single package. This process helps remove changes from the limelight and external influences (Brown 1990).

The expansion of the issue network associated with health policy has provided resources to use in developing new policy approaches. That network has grown both inside and outside of government. As Morone (1990a) points out, the extragovernment growth in the network has been induced by government programs, particularly those that mandated citizen participation and those that funded external evaluation research. The general concession of the domestic agenda to Congress has helped accelerate the growth in health policy experts in Congress, including some who focus on particular issues as Albert Gore has done with organ transplantation (Mueller 1989) and some who cast their nets much more broadly, such as Henry Waxman and Edward Kennedy. Those individuals have expanded their staffs to include more in-house health policy expertise, and they have become active members of issue networks that include experts outside of government.

These optimistic perspectives on the environment for changes in health policy should not be interpreted as arguments for the inevitability of national health insurance. Several members of the health policy issue network remain disappointed that we do not yet have national health insurance, and they are quite pessimistic about the prospects (Ginzberg 1990). We can continue to expect great difficulty in making fundamental trade-offs to achieve particular public objectives. Ginzberg has articulated this problem vis-à-vis adopting the Canadian system:

> The same public that admires the Canadian system also expresses a deep desire for more and better health care services. Even a schizophrenic public that wants both effective cost containment and more and better health care services appreciates, at least intuitively, that effective cost controls will result in less, not more, desirable and desired services. Accordingly, Americans are slow to lobby for basic health care reforms that might result in an effective cap on the amount of money that flows into the health care system. (p. 1465)

As I have argued throughout this book, incremental solutions to specific problems will often generate new, and sometimes more serious, problems.

The prospects for continued incremental adjustments are quite favorable. The chances of seeing any comprehensive policy enacted are considerably less. Although there is increasing agreement that more dramatic change is needed, there is no consensus as to what that change should be. The window of opportunity for major change is opening, as evident in public sentiment, but no particular idea to accomplish that change is as yet the idea sweeping across the land that would provide the obvious solution awaiting congressional enactment.

SPECIFIC SUGGESTIONS FOR REFORM IN THE 1990S

Many specific proposals to expand access to health care were introduced in the 102d Congress in 1991. The renewed interest in various comprehensive health care acts is impressive. There have been national health plans suggested in previous sessions of Congress, but activity accelerated following the release of the Pepper Commission report. Members of Congress are more sensitized now to the problems facing millions of Americans who lack health insurance. In addition, millions of Americans with insurance are concerned that the cost of insurance premiums will become prohibitive and that they may lose access to health insurance. These are concerns policymakers will want to address. Current proposals to reform the health care system focus on changing the way health care is financed, with little attention paid to how it is delivered, or to the distribution of services. With the legislative attention focused on finance, two concerns are addressed in most proposals—how to assure access to health insurance and how to contain total health care expenditures. Some proposals include provisions related to the quality of health care services. Others address issues concerning the availability of health care services in underserved geographic areas.

Health care reform proposals in the 1990s can be grouped into three general categories; play-or-pay, voucher, and single-payer. These categories array various plans according to the source of funding for health insurance. They also imply variation in how health care costs are reimbursed.

The play-or-pay approach builds on the existing system of providing insurance through employers. In this scheme, employers would be required to either provide health insurance for employees and their dependents or pay into a public fund that would be used to subsidize the costs associated with individually purchased health insurance. Proposals adopting this approach define employer groups as all employers of a certain size purchasing insurance from a given company. Within those groups, variations in premium charges would be limited. This is a strategy to keep premiums affordable. Another approach is to require that all insurance premiums in a given community be the same, which is called *community rating*. Because the purpose of reforming the private insurance market is to make insurance affordable to small employers, measures such as those just described are thought to be necessary. They prevent charging small employers high premiums based on the adverse experiences of a single employee in a single firm.

In the play-or-pay approach, the public sector would organize a single plan for employees whose employers chose to pay rather than offer health insurance. In effect, a large group is created whose insurance premiums are based on a group rate subsidized by the government. This approach will provide financial access to all those who are currently employed. Various definitions of employment are included in these proposals, ranging from fifteen to thirty-five hours per week. Access to health insurance, without other changes to reach the uninsured who are unemployed, would not be universal. Millions of Americans currently without insurance, however, would be insured under the plan.

Employers who currently do not offer health insurance would see increases in business costs. The hope of proponents of this approach is that there would be a level playing field, offering no single employer a special advantage. A variation on the play-or-pay proposal is to require that all employers provide health insurance, as is done in Hawaii. A minimum benefits package for health insurance is specified in proposals to assure that catastrophic expenses are covered.

The voucher approach to reform relies on individual decisions to purchase health insurance. Tax credits are offered to offset the costs of health insurance, and for the poorest citizens, the credits are issued in advance as vouchers with which to purchase insurance. Proposals to create tax incentives sometimes include requirements that specify the minimum benefits that must be included in all insurance plans. They may also include provisions requiring community rating.

The single-payer approach comes closest to resembling the Canadian system. All persons would be insured by the same payer, either government directly or government through a third party. This parallels the Medicare program currently offered to the nation's elderly. Medicare payments are made through fiscal intermediaries, private insurance companies. Those companies are responsible for administering the program according to regulations written and enforced by the government. In the single-payer model, the same approach would be used for all Americans, not just those over the age of sixty-five. Eligibility for insurance would be based on citizenship and/or legal status, not employment or income. Most single-payer proposals require extensive government financing and therefore specify new sources of revenue. Conceptually, though, it is possible to adopt a single-payer approach while retaining a premium structure that places the burden of financing on those enrolled rather than on a taxing system.

A variety of cost-containment provisions are included in proposals to reform health care financing. The most common provisions are those that continue the prospective payment system (PPS) and implement the resource-based relative-value system (RBRVS) to pay physicians. Many proposals also incorporate aggregate limits on all health care expenditures. Some proposals suggest controls over the supply of health care facilities and technology, whereas others create special commissions in each state responsible for state plans that determine limits on capital expansion. A small number of proposals, usually those adopting the single-payer approach, rely on direct negotiations between government and providers to control total expenditures. Other proposals, usually those adopting a voucher approach, rely on a competitive marketplace and wise consumer choices to control costs. None of the proposals offers a new magic bullet guaranteed to control health care expenditures.

Reform proposals offered in the early 1990s are generally silent on issues related to quality of care. Many proposals support continuing and expanding efforts to develop practice guidelines. As summarized in the discussion in chapter 5, these proposals are often attempts to control costs, not assure quality of care. Some proposals reform the legal system that considers malpractice cases, but again with cost control rather than quality as the objective. The most favorable provisions related to quality care are those that create new benefits and/or programs for preventive care. Once again, though, the proposals submitted in Congress have very little to offer. Many of them include provisions for well-baby care, prenatal care, and screening for cancers (mammography benefits are quite common). Very few though, carry the philosophy of preventive care to the logical extension of benefits to finance wellness programs, nutritional education, and smoking cessation.

The obvious question is: How likely is it that any of these bills will pass? The prospects in 1992 were quite dim, especially for any legislation that requires federal spending. Provisions of a budget compromise struck between members of Congress and President Bush in 1990 require that any new spending be balanced by reductions in the same category of budgeting. For example, any increases in spending within social programs such as Medicare and Medicaid must be matched with spending reductions in other social programs. Having enacted several incremental measures to expand access to care in recent years, Congress may well want to observe the changes induced by those efforts before moving forward with other suggestions, a "period of oversight," as Paul Rettig, an officer of the American Hospital Association, has said (Cooper 1991).

Submitting legislation in 1991 and 1992 though, may have been a preliminary step toward more dramatic change later. If a number of observers are correct in reading the political tea leaves, the American public increasingly favors fundamental change in the health care system. By introducing legislation in 1991–92 members of Congress initiated further debate and research on important policy ideas in preparation for the time when the window of opportunity opens wide and a national plan can be adopted. In the interim, we should witness an intensifying debate about some of the key elements of such a plan, including: how to generate revenues to pay for a national plan, how to pay medical care providers, what services to include in a plan, what criteria to use in determining eligibility for benefits, and how to administer any new program.

The prospect for some reform of health care financing during the four-year presidential term beginning in 1993 would appear to be quite good. President Clinton emphasized the need for health care reform during his campaign and continues to call for change. He has linked the crisis in health care finance to the more general, and some would argue more serious, problem with the national economy. Health care costs plague American businesses, and families cannot achieve financial security unless they have health insurance. Although we may not yet know precisely what the health care delivery and finance system will be in the next millennium, we can be more confident than ever that it will be different.

The inauguration of President Clinton, combined with legislation introduced late in the 102d Congress, has given rise to one more variation in reform proposals—managed competition. The president advocates creating regional networks in every state that would negotiate with insurance plans to provide, at a minimum, basic benefits for all citizens in that region for the same premium (variations would be allowed only for age and family size). This reform could be combined with an employer mandate or could evolve into a single-payer approach.

Although the prospects for national reform are still unpredictable, actions are already being taken by state governments. During 1992, twelve states began planning for innovative changes, with the planning financed by the Robert Wood Johnson Foundation. Florida has initiated a new program aimed at increasing insurance availability for children by offering health insurance through the schools. Minnesota has begun a new program to finance care for the uninsured by taxing providers of care. We can expect further experimentation by states as they both try to contain the costs of the Medicaid program and yet provide greater financial access to care.

Conclusion

A growing consensus is emerging that the health care delivery system in the United States needs radical reform. There is as yet, however, no overwhelming consensus that defines the specifics of that reform. To be successful, radical policy solutions will need the support of the key players in the issue network, including the president, influential members of Congress, and the various professional groups who would be expected to abide by a new set of rules. Not all parties need to agree to the same plan before legislation to reform the system would pass, but the key players in the issue network must be on board. At a minimum, that group includes the president and committee and party leaders in Congress. The views of the latter are influenced by interest groups who can influence electoral outcomes, so they too must agree with the planks in any legislation before it would become reality.

There have been moments in the history of health care policy when many pundits believed the United States was close to adopting a national health insurance scheme. Medicare is a form of insurance for the elderly and can be viewed as a precursor to national health insurance for all. During the presidency of Richard Nixon, several of the most influential political actors in the issue network supported national health insurance: the president, the chairperson of the Ways and Means Committee in the House of Representatives, and the chairperson of the Labor and Human Resources Committee in the Senate. The Watergate affair crippled the Nixon presidency, however, and the Tidal Basin incident (a stripper was seen with Wilbur Mills) ended the political career of the Ways and Means chair. Nonetheless, hope for a national system remained alive during the 1970s, and the Health Planning Act of that decade was seen by some as a means of rendering the delivery system more rational in preparation for a national plan.

During the late 1970s and the Jimmy Carter presidency, a president once again supported national health insurance, as did the chair of the Senate Labor and Human Resources Committee (Senator Kennedy). The plans were quite different, however, and the Carter presidency was doomed to ineffectiveness in efforts to work with Congress.

A new dawn has sprung for those who advocate national health care reform. The continued escalation of health expenditures and the increased number of Americans without any health insurance coverage have combined to create an environment conducive to at least seriously considering reform of the system. When analysts and politicians compare the performance of the U.S. health care delivery system with those of other Western nations, they are dismayed that the United States spends more (controlling for population and currency value) than other nations while not performing as well on such health indicators as infant mortality. Those comparative data have precipitated the question, why can't we be more like them?

The answer is that our political and social systems are not like theirs. Instead of a corporatist approach to resolving public policy issues, the U.S. system is characterized by decentralized and fragmented decision-making structures. Instead of an acceptance of government intervention as necessary to secure the welfare of all, the U.S. cultural expectation is one of minimal government intervention designed only to protect the welfare of a few. Changes can and undoubtedly will occur in the U.S. approach to financing health care, but the changes will be incremental in nature until incremental solutions have proved ineffective.

8

. . .

The Future
of Health Care Policy in
the United States

By the turn of the next century, the pattern of organizing, delivering, and financing health care in the United States could be radically different from the approaches used in the 1980s. Throughout the early 1990s, policies have been adopted that appear to signal major shifts in the traditional norms that have guided previous policies. The national government adopted more restrictive payment policies that influence how health care is delivered. Prospective payment policies in the Medicare program encouraged an increased use of outpatient and ambulatory care, and relative-value–based reimbursement of physicians' services reduced the financial advantage long enjoyed by specialists over primary care providers.

The debate of the 1990s is the question of how extensive government influence on medical care delivery should become. State governments have entered that debate with policies designed to restrict the expansion of medical care facilities and changes in licensing and regulations to permit more use of allied health professionals and different uses of health care facilities. The national government began the 1990s by extending the influence of government more directly into the practice of medicine. The Omnibus Reconciliation Act of 1989 created the new Agency for Health Care Policy and Research, whose mission includes developing practice guidelines to determine optimal medical treatment responses to certain health conditions.

Despite pressures to reduce government spending in both the states and the nation, the 1990s is a time of increased government activism in health policy. As described in the early chapters of this book, many problems associated with delivering and financing medical care have become more visible in recent years. There has never been a time when all U.S. citizens were covered by health insurance, but the number without coverage has increased dramatically since the mid-1980s and continues to climb. Geographical access problems in rural areas became more obvious following the implementation of prospective payment in the Medicare program. Questions concerning the quality of care became more substantial after small area research revealed wide variations in the practice of medicine. Publicity surrounding these issues has increased in the 1990s, and the pressure for policy responses has intensified. Responses have been somewhat constrained because of the crisis created by the federal budget deficit and similar difficulties in many of the states. Nonetheless, government officials have reacted with the policies described throughout this book. Now the question is What further policy developments should we expect?

Any answers would have to be conjectural. Using the framework developed in this book, we can at least develop informed and logical guesses. Two approaches are used in this chapter. First, developments in each of the three pillars of health policy (cost containment, access, and quality) are examined in order to forecast the next logical incremental steps. Second, changes in the issue network are reviewed with an eye toward predicting the likelihood of more dramatic action. Finally, the book will close with a discussion of U.S. national health care policy in the context of global developments.

Developments in Health Policies

Health policy in the United States is a complex mosaic of particular policies enacted to resolve what are perceived to be specific deficiencies in the exchange between providers and consumers. Government is involved directly in that exchange when the consumers are insured under public programs such as Medicare and Medicaid. When there is no direct involvement, there remains a public interest to protect because, as argued in the first chapter, adequate health care is necessary to enable citizens to pursue their inherent rights. Pursuant to that public interest, government will act to protect consumers from fraud and poor quality care. Government intervention can also be expected when access to care is denied, keeping some citizens from a full range of opportunities. Finally, government can be expected to act in its own behalf to lower the costs of health care. All actions will be in response to specific problems and are most likely to be based on previous government efforts. Such is the nature of incremental policymaking.

PROTECTING QUALITY

Initial forays into assuring the quality of care were designed to prevent quackery and establish minimum qualifications for persons in the health care professions. Licensing health professionals and defining their scope of practice remain critical policy concerns. The number of health professions has grown, and the potential for overlap exists. Each profession attempts to claim its own special expertise and jealously guards their turf against the intrusion of other professions when attempts are made to alter scopes of practice. Cost-containment and access concerns complicate state policymaking on issues of professional practice (health professional licensing and scope of practice are state policies). Certain allied health professionals are trained to perform many functions that only a couple of decades ago were the exclusive purview of physicians. Nurse practitioners and physicians' assistants can complete physical examinations and perform many of the routine diagnostic and treatment functions of primary care physicians. Allied health professionals are less costly to consumers, and may be willing to practice in geographic shortage areas that have not attracted physicians.

Policies have been enacted expanding the scope of practice of nurse practitioners, physicians' assistants, and other professionals. Lucrative funding is available for rural health clinics through federal policies that require that they use allied professionals. The allied professionals themselves, though, want more. As the number of physicians' assistants increases, many of them specialize by assisting surgeons and other specialist physicians. Nurses insist that four years of undergraduate training is a starting point (rather than a terminal degree for registered nurses) and that more postgraduate training should be offered. Specialization among the allied professionals is likely to create further conflict with physicians and diminish the value of the allied professionals for policy objectives related to cost containment and access. Health care expenditures represent an ever larger share of the nation's wealth, and we should expect battles to intensify among groups wanting a share of that wealth. State governments will spend much of the next decade sorting out the respective responsibilities (scope of practice) of health professionals.

Health professionals will continue to press for legislative relief from the costly burden of malpractice litigation. Physicians view costs associated with malpractice actions (insurance premiums, jury awards, and defensive medicine) as one the two leading causes of health care price inflation (Taylor, Leitman, and Edwards 1991). Consumers need protection from wrongful action by physicians, but the current state of affairs exceeds reasonable standards. When the recourse used affects more than the actions targeted, change is in order. State governments can be expected to continue reforming malpractice statutes.

In the delivery of any service, quality is normally assessed by comparing real actions against "gold standards." In medical care, the standards have historically been moving targets—medicine has been as much (if not more) art as science. Therefore, it has been difficult to question the judgment of individual physicians. The increase in malpractice litigation, combined with the results of small area analysis, have established precedence for believing there are certain norms that can be applied to all physicians' practices. They are as yet, however, ill defined. Now that the mystique of the all-knowing physician has been cracked, efforts to develop more precise practice standards are accelerating. The medical community has long been interested in improving the practice of medicine, and research articles in such journals as *The New England Journal of Medicine* and *Journal of the American Medical Association* have assisted in those efforts. In addition to the traditional means of improving medical practice through scientific research within the medical community, the 1980s and early 1990s saw the advent of using health services research for that purpose. Scholars trained in statistical analysis used data collected concerning diagnostic and treatment decisions to compare decisions across physicians' practices. Individual physicians' decisions could also be judged as appropriate or inappropriate by panels of specialists. This analysis includes the assessment of differences in outcomes that result as a consequence of treatment decisions. Comparisons are made among treatment decisions, based on cost and outcomes.

Policy implications of the trend toward external analysis of physicians' decisions are already apparent. Professional review organizations (PROS) are used by the Medicare program to judge the appropriateness of hospital admissions and length of stays in hospitals. Administrators in Medicaid programs routinely review the appropriateness of treatment regimens, relying on medical directors and pharmaceutical experts for advice. Private firms now market utilization review services as cost savings programs. Although many of these efforts are enacted in the name of cost containment, they are at least subtle challenges to the quality of care being rendered also.

The next incremental step in policies related to quality of care has been initiated. The federal government has begun an effort to set practice guidelines that all physicians can follow, given a certain set of conditions present in patients.

Once those guidelines are set, they are likely to be linked to reimbursement policies and used in malpractice litigation. The federal government will develop and disseminate medical practice guidelines, intensifying policy debates about the quality of medical care.

The fact that over thirty-three million Americans do not have any health care insurance is reason to expect at least some suggestions for public policy response. At least as many Americans who are insured nonetheless face high medical expenses, either because insurance policies do not include payment for routine care or because insurance premiums have become quite expensive. Continuous publicity about the plight of particular American families who have lost health insurance benefits intensifies the pressure on elected officials to act. The federal government has expanded financial access by adding categories of eligibility to the Medicaid program, especially for children in families earning less than poverty-level incomes. Those measures have only slowed the growth in the uninsured population.

Many of the most publicized cases of uninsurance involve families with a full-time worker in the household. The stereotypical image of families being insured through the workplace does not hold under empirical scrutiny. Most of the general public is quite sympathetic to the plight of hard-working families, so resolving their social problems is a desirable function for government. We should expect state and federal policies in the next few years that either facilitate (through tax benefits) or mandate insurance availability from all employers.

Will government go all the way and guarantee financial access for all citizens through a system of national health insurance? The previous chapter considered this question and the reply was vague. Some may argue that the country is close to a national system of financing care, but the most compelling evidence, based on an analysis of public opinion, concludes that the political will is not yet in place (Blendon and Edwards 1991). Public support for change is general and not yet overwhelming for any particular reform. Nonetheless, momentum is building, and the interim incremental policies are not likely to resolve the problem of financial access for all citizens. Therefore we should expect the state and federal governments to continue considering government financing for all medical care but without enacting a comprehensive program in the near future.

179

Even when consumers are able to pay for health care, it may not be available in their communities. This book used the plight of rural communities to illustrate this condition, but many of the nation's inner cities exhibit similar problems. Large public institutions in those communities are overwhelmed with low-income patients and persons with AIDS. Overcrowded hospital emergency rooms can no longer serve as a primary care provider of last resort for the poor. The states and the federal government have passed changes in Medicaid and Medicare reimbursement policies to redress payment inequities vis-à-vis rural and inner city hospitals. The states have changed licensure statutes to allow more flexibility and innovation in designing health care delivery institutions. Other policies provide incentives to providers locating in underserved areas and to institutions willing to change the configuration of the services they offer.

Access continues to be a problem in many communities, in part because the policies enacted since 1983 have focused on narrowly defined elements of the delivery system. We have not had a unified strategy of reforming the system based on a policy of integrated services. Since the diminution of health planning in the early 1980s, we have been approaching the access problem on a piecemeal basis, one group, one type of geographic location, and one type of service at a time. New programs, including a federal program to integrate networks of rural hospitals, are reinstating health planning practices. We should expect additional state and national policies that incorporate principles of health planning into efforts to guarantee and expand access to medical care services in underserved areas.

COST-CONTAINMENT POLICIES

No other aspect of health care policy has received more attention during the past ten years than efforts to contain increases in health care expenditures. The federal government in particular has been active, since Medicare expenditures are a significant percent of all federal expenditures and therefore a leading target for budget savings. State governments will undoubtedly begin to view Medicaid expenditures in a similar manner.

Two major policy initiatives enacted by the federal government have targeted first hospital and then physicians' services for price controls. Prospective payment and resource-based relative-value scales have not been labeled as price controls, but they do constrain the prices the federal government will pay for services rendered to Medicare clients. Evidence presented earlier in this book demonstrated the effectiveness of the hospital policies in reducing increases in inpatient expenditures. Hospital expenditures, however, have continued to escalate. Two shifts have occurred—from inpatient to outpatient charges and from Medicare to other sources of payment. Controls on physicians' expenditures may prove to be more effective since the basis is more encompassing. There are no shifts comparable to the inpatient-outpatient movement in hospital services and charges. There is a potential shift of sorts, however, from high prices per service to higher volume of services at lower prices. By addressing only one aspect of health care delivery at a time, public policies are vulnerable to the types of circumvention just described. Incremental policies to affect a specific behavior, such as hospital inpatient charges or physician charges for specific services, can be quite effective and yet not have the desired impact on total health care expenditures.

Expenditures are a function of the price of services times the quantity of services delivered. Most policies enacted to date have focused on the price of services. Policymakers are understandably reluctant to consider restricting the quantity of services, fearful of interpretations that they are sacrificing quality of care at the altar of cost containment. Increased debate about the right to die and the value of life-extending services provides an opportunity to begin discussions of limiting reimbursable services. Government officials will remain reluctant to impose regulations restricting services, but Medicare policies can encourage consideration of limits. As of 1 December 1991, all hospitals, nursing homes, and health maintenance organizations receiving Medicare payments must inform patients of their right to refuse care that prolongs life in a persistent vegetative state, that is, their right to sign and present a living will and/or a durable power of attorney designating someone else to decide if treatment should continue.

The federal government is unlikely to adopt a rigid policy of rationing care in order to contain expenditures, but the effort under way in Oregon may be repeated in other states. States are more constrained in spending in that they are constitutionally forbidden to end a given fiscal year in debt. Therefore, others may want to copy Oregon's approach to paying for only those services the state budget can afford. Activity of this type will most likely involve policies that do not require federal approval, given the difficulty encountered by Oregon (the request for a waiver of Medicaid rules was rejected by the Bush administration in August 1992). State governments can be expected to experiment with various means of containing Medicaid expenditures in the next ten years, absent a federal policy to pay for all health care.

The federal government is likely to continue adopting incremental policies that first focus on controlling prices charged and then begin considering policies that constrain the quantity of services. On the price front, the federal government is likely to expand price controls to more dimensions of health care delivery, including prescription medications (funded by Medicare), outpatient hospital services, and psychiatric care. On the quantity front, the federal government is likely to use practice guidelines as leverage in a scheme to deny payment for unnecessary services.

INTEGRATION OF THEMES: THE CASE OF AIDS

Policy responses to the AIDS epidemic are indicative of how the three themes of cost containment, access, and quality of care must be integrated. An ongoing concern is to control the spread of the disease. This public health issue involves providing access to educational and preventive services. Rather than waiting for those in need to initiate contact, however, the emphasis is to reach them with services whether or not they choose to make contact. Prevention is a concern not often expressed in public policies targeted to reforming the health care delivery system, but the special case of AIDS illustrates the cost of ignoring preventive measures.

More typical access concerns are included in AIDS policy deliberations. Persons with AIDS (PWAS) are sometimes denied access to services because of an unfounded fear that the infection will spread. Regulatory policies and conditions of participation in public programs can influence provider behavior to assure access to care for PWAS. Access to care is also a problem because many of the PWAS are unable to purchase private insurance. They are likely lose their employment but remain alive beyond any postemployment insurance benefit. Policymakers in the states, under provisions of federal legislation, are investigating ways of providing insurance to this population.

The financial access problem is related to issues of cost containment. Caring for PWAS in the final months of their lives can be very expensive, as high as $50,000 per case and an average of $32,000 per year per patient (Hellinger 1991). Policymakers will need to consider policies that lower the cost of treatment by promoting the use of hospices and finding more cost-effective means of treatment.

Issues regarding quality of care arise in treating PWAS because of U.S. policies governing the development and marketing of new drugs. Extensive testing and retesting is required before drugs can be made available to the general public. In the special case of AIDS, though, those delays can deny a thread of hope in an otherwise hopeless situation. Congress has in recent years addressed this problem by speeding the time for drug approval and permitting exceptions for AIDS as a terminal condition. New medicines that add to the life expectancy of PWAS add to the costs involved in a lifetime treatment of the condition. They are also beyond the means of many PWAS to purchase. In this single dimension of improving quality through new treatment we can see the problems created for cost containment and access to care.

Finally, treating PWAS in some of the nation's large cities has created stress for health care facilities that treat the poor. In New York City, for example, the increased number of AIDS patients in public hospitals is creating crowded conditions and constraining the ability of those institutions to continue to provide care to all comers. When the health care system has to deal with a crisis such as AIDS that requires intensive use of resources, the weaknesses in its safety-net services are exposed. This special problem has, in summary, demonstrated the need for policymakers to consider issues of cost containment, access, and quality simultaneously.

SUMMARY

By examining current and recent policies, we can confidently predict future policies. They are likely to be incremental extensions of previous activities. Only if the political climate changes drastically should we expect anything other than incremental change. Two circumstances could change the environment: a different configuration of the issue network or cataclysmic events that require nonincremental response. The latter could be either a single event, such as an epidemic affecting all segments of the population, or a series of events, such as repeated market failures in particular industries. Elements of both sets of circumstances can be identified in the U.S. policy environment for health policy, but they are as yet still insufficient to produce dramatic change.

Changes in the Issue Network

There have been important changes in the issue network in health policy. The network began expanding in the 1970s and continues to grow now. Just as the dollars spent on health care escalate and employment in the health care industry grows, the number of analysts trained to examine health policy issues grows. Many of those analysts are finding employment in the offices of U.S. senators and representatives, state legislators, the federal bureaucracy, and state bureaucracies. In those positions they develop suggestions for new policies or, more likely, modifications of ongoing efforts. In part as a result of their efforts, more legislators in the federal and state governments are focusing their attention on health care issues.

The expansion of the issue network within legislative bodies results in more opportunities to initiate new policies. The initiatives are likely to be focused on particular pieces of the total mosaic of government health policies, because each legislator has focused on his or her special interest within the broader context. The key sources of power to accomplish sweeping change remain the same—certain committee chairpersons and the chief executive. In Congress, the majority leader of the Senate and the speaker of the House join this smaller circle of important players in the issue network.

The influence of interest groups within the network has changed in recent years. During the 1960s and 1970s, the power of organized medicine was assumed to reign supreme in health policy debates. During the 1980s, the ability of organized medicine to thwart public policy diminished. Adopting prospective payment for hospital reimbursement was the first strong signal that the issue network was no longer monolithic, under the control of organized medicine. The decade of the 1980s closed with Congress adopting a new reimbursement scheme for physicians, under which there will be winners and losers in the medical profession. Although this policy was ultimately accepted by organized medicine, it passed because the power of that particular group had eroded.

Why has the influence of organized medicine declined? There are two general explanations. First, the nearly twenty-year focus on cost containment as a public policy objective drew attention to the health professions and their incomes. Second, the growth in health care expenditures made this a policy arena attracting the attention of many groups, expanding the issue network at the expense of entrenched groups.

The policy environment drew attention to the high costs of health care during the 1970s. Policymakers during the second half of that decade were willing to trust in the voluntary efforts of health care providers to reduce increases in their charges. By the early 1980s, the voluntary efforts had failed and policymakers realized that they would have to impose financial discipline on providers. By that time, much of the explosion in the number of health care analysts in Congress and the executive branch had occurred and there were experts capable of challenging the substantive arguments offered by health care professionals. More importantly, health services researchers had contributed thorough analyses of hospital charges and a scheme for prospectively pricing hospital services. Later the research community was able to contribute a well-crafted scheme for reimbursing physicians based on the time spent with patients and the skills required to complete particular diagnoses and treatments.

A set of circumstances had come together to change the nature of the issue network and the direction of public policy. Previous policies had been declared failures in light of increasing health expenditures. An infusion of analytical talent had changed the comparative advantage of health professionals when discussing the complicated substance of health care policies. Finally, when the window of opportunity opened because of the first two conditions, the research community was ready with proposals for change.

Milestones have been reached with new reimbursement policies, but two grim realities remain. First, the impacts on health expenditures have been real but minor. The overall pace of increase continues virtually unabated and still represents a serious policy problem. Second, other issues have arisen in the 1990s that challenge the abilities of the issue network, namely how to provide medical care to over thirty-three million uninsured Americans. These issues would appear to challenge the political system to devise solutions beyond the normal incremental adjustments we have come to expect—and beyond the piecemeal approach of addressing one of the three objectives (quality, access, cost containment) at a time.

National Health Insurance?

Policy discussions in the United States increasingly include suggestions to adopt a system of national health insurance. The suggestions range from incentives encouraging employers to provide insurance to a single system, financed and administered by the federal government. For the purposes of this discussion, national health insurance (NHI) will mean a single system created by federal legislation, funded and administered by some combination of state and federal sources.

Some actors within the issue network advocate a government takeover of all responsibilities for health insurance in the United States. Several large American corporations have argued that providing access to health care is a social responsibility more properly addressed by government than by employers. Further, providing health care insurance through the workplace, when other nations do so through government plans, places American corporations at a competitive disadvantage in the world marketplace. Although somewhat persuasive, this position is not universally advocated by all American corporations. Many of them assume that providing health insurance coverage is a means of offering benefits as part of an attractive compensation package that helps in recruiting and retaining workers. Thus, the corporate community does not speak as a single voice in the issue network.

Organized labor, on the other hand, has consistently advocated a scheme of national health insurance. An independent source of health insurance benefits would make workers less dependent on employers, which in turn creates more possibilities for labor stoppage when deemed necessary. Further, removing health insurance benefits from the compensation package may create opportunities to negotiate higher salaries. Not all workers, however, favor NHI. Many oppose it because of their distrust of government programs. Others do not want to lose the tax advantages of receiving some compensation in the form of health insurance premium payments that are not included in taxable income. Finally, some oppose NHI based on the tax burden it would create. Labor organizations may favor NHI, but their influence within the issue network is mitigated by dissension in the ranks.

Organized medicine has long opposed NHI. Some groups within the medical community, though, now advocate more intrusive government programs. For them, government programs can address both financial and service needs. Financially, patients without health insurance present a problem in collecting payment for services rendered. As the numbers of uninsured continue to grow, providers are increasingly likely to be treating those persons. Therefore, securing a source of payment for them is in the providers' best interest. Providers also recognize that persons without health insurance are not receiving adequate health care services because of financial barriers to access. This is especially troubling when the uninsured include large numbers of children; hence, the American Academy of Pediatrics advocates a national system to replace Medicaid. Although many provider groups, including the American Medical Association, advocate reform of the current system of health care finance, they all stop short of advocating universal and comprehensive national health insurance. There are, however, some providers who do advocate NHI. Among those is an organization of physicians, although at the present time they do not speak for an organized majority of all physicians. Organized medicine is not uniformly opposed to reform, but does speak out against suggestions which would dramatically reduce physician income.

Elected officials are another group with split opinion on this issue. Of the myriad proposals suggested in the 102d Congress, few were comprehensive

NHI. Most proposals contained the typical incremental suggestions for an expansion of existing mechanisms to cover more of the uninsured. Most common were suggestions to expand the employment-based availability of health insurance by either creating tax incentives or enacting mandates that would compel all employers (with a very few exceptions) to provide health insurance. Some proposals contained provisions to expand Medicaid eligibility to reach more of the poor without full-time employment, and others created new categories of eligibility for Medicare coverage. A few proposals envisioned a unified system of insurance under government sponsorship. These proposals would have the federal government establish minimum benefits standards and have each state responsible for universal coverage within its borders.

Financing for the systems would be a blend of payroll taxes, taxes on such goods as cigarettes and alcohol, and premiums paid by the insured. A single schedule of reimbursement for all health care services would be established under these plans. Only under these comprehensive plans would there be a prospect of attacking simultaneously problems in quality, cost containment, and access. The network of policymakers influential in health care, though, is not united in support in any of these plans. President Bush did not advocate any policy to address access issues until the pressures of the 1992 presidential campaign moved him to do so in January 1992. There is a voice for NHI among policymakers in the issue network, but no strong consensus.

Analysts within the network have assisted in developing the incremental policies of recent years and contribute to the NHI debate by defining the impacts of various reform proposals. They have also identified certain weaknesses in the current system for financing health care, most particularly the costs of administration associated with relying on a complex mix of sources of fee structures and payment. Analysts have also identified the wide variation in medical practice styles and the costs associated with that phenomenon. Analysts have not, however, come any closer than others in the issue network to a consensus about what an ideal NHI system would be.

Overall, NHI is on the policy agenda and has advocates within the issue network. There are no opponents to NHI who threaten to block any and all initiatives. The network has grown beyond ceding that type of veto power to health professionals (especially the AMA). There is not as yet, however, sufficient agreement among members of the network to support NHI and see it enacted.

Conclusion

The United States remains one of only two Western nations without a national system of insuring access to quality medical care for all its citizens. Does that mean we are the villains of the world? Hardly. The U.S. health care system is, for those with access, the most technologically advanced care available anywhere for those who can afford it. Medical research has long been supported in this country, both privately and publicly. As a result the U.S. medical community has developed the most advanced diagnostic and treatment procedures possible. Medical education in the United States is unsurpassed in providing training to professionals who want to use the latest and most advanced techniques.

The strengths of the U.S. health care delivery system generate its weaknesses. Using the latest developments in medical care technology and well-trained specialists is the most expensive means possible to provide care to patients, making the U.S. system the most costly in the world. Training medical students in the latest techniques in an environment that includes access to all the advanced equipment they could want and to faculty role models in specialized medicine produces students with little interest in primary care. It is also an expensive model for medical education, which means that after paying large amounts of money for training, physicians want to recoup those costs through charges to patients. High patient charges make it difficult for insurance companies to provide benefits at low costs, driving the costs of insurance up and in many cases beyond the capacities of small groups and individuals to pay.

The medical care model evident in our large teaching institutions is one in which specialists and expensive diagnostic equipment are readily available. Such is not the case in rural medical practices, making those practices less than desirable to many medical school graduates. New reimbursement systems based on average costs make it difficult for rural hospitals with few patients to survive financially if even one of them exceeds the average. Other public policies, enacted with the best of intentions, affect some institutions disproportionately and adversely. For example, as per provisions of a 1991 statute, patients are to be informed of their rights related to self-determination by all hospitals, health maintenance organizations, and nursing homes. Those rights include the right to sign living wills. The purpose of the law is to assure that all patients are able to refuse treatment that merely prolongs life without improving the quality of life. If an elderly patient already concerned about adverse consequences of the least intrusive procedure, however, is informed of such rights, he or she may become overly concerned about the prospects of dying, triggering psychosomatic illness and depression. This problem can in turn be addressed by a staff social worker, but small rural institutions are unlikely to have such assistance available.

The problems we confront in U.S. health care policy exist because policymakers have not adopted comprehensive approaches when establishing government policies. Instead, a single issue has been approached at any given time, and even then not all dimensions of that issue have been considered when developing specific policies. The prospective payment system was adopted after a thorough examination of national data and testing in New Jersey. Neither of those sources of analysis could reveal the impact of the new system on individual small rural hospitals. During the late 1980s and early 1990s Congress had to devote considerable legislative effort to fixing the problems PPS created for those institutions. Effective cost-containment policy adversely affected access in rural communities.

The health planning legislation of 1974 was the last major attempt by the federal government to develop comprehensive policy. Since that time, legislative efforts have been specific to issues in cost containment (PPS, relative-value scales), access (outreach programs in rural areas), and quality (creating the AHCPR and calling for practice guidelines). The United States lags considerably behind other nations that have national systems. Other nations, though, look to the United States for effective solutions to particular problems, such as determining fair prices for medical care services. The United States has devoted considerable energies to developing effective micro-level policies, whereas other nations have developed macro-level systems that now appear to need some micro-level solutions to their problems, particularly in cost containment. The Canadian government is experiencing fiscal pressures caused by escalating health care costs, as are the British. Those countries are examining U.S. policies for possible solutions at the same time that analysts in the United States are examining their systems in hopes of discovering the nirvana for a national system. The result is convergence: "Great Britain and the United States appear to be converging on a point at which our health care systems may look very similar" (Vall-Spinosa 1991).

We might be disappointed that the United States faces severe problems, including the millions of uninsured who have less than adequate access to health care, but we should also be pleased that in our incremental way we have gained a greater appreciation of the costs and quality of medical decisions. Policymakers in the United States may be avoiding the future problems of cost containment by addressing that issue before adopting a national system.

The best public policy will emerge from an understanding of the interactions of public actions and private sector responses in health care delivery. By focusing attention narrowly on specific problems, members of the issue network have gained an appreciation for and understanding of that interaction. During the next twenty years, U.S. policymakers face the even greater challenge of integrating the set of policies enacted to address specific objectives into a single approach that satisfies the goal of access to quality care at reasonable costs.

• • •

References

Aaron, H. J. 1991. *Serious and Unstable Condition: Financing America's Health Care*. Washington, D.C.: The Brookings Institution.

Aaron, H. J., and W. B. Schwartz. 1984. *The Painful Prescription: Rationing Hospital Care*. Washington, D.C.: The Brookings Institution.

Adrian, C. 1985. *Social Policies in Western Industrial Societies*. Berkeley: University of California Press.

Aiken, L. H. 1989. "The Hospital Nursing Shortage: A Paradox of Increasing Supply and Increasing Vacancy Rates." *Western Journal of Medicine* 151 (July): 87–92.

Alford, R. R. 1975. *Health Care Politics: Ideology and Interest Group Barriers to Reform*. Chicago: University of Chicago Press.

Alston, C. 1989. "Belt-Tightening in Medicare Pits Doctor vs. Doctor." *Congressional Quarterly* (7 October): 2605–9.

American Hospital Association. 1987. *Profile of Small or Rural Hospitals 1980–1986*. Chicago: American Hospital Association.

———. 1988. *Hospital Statistics*. 1987 edition. Chicago: American Hospital Association.

———. 1991. *Hospital Statistics* 1991–92 edition. Chicago: American Hospital Association.

Associated Press. 1990. "Medical-Benefit Expenses Up, Consultants Say." *Omaha World Herald* (30 January): 21.

Austen, W. G. 1988. Statement of the American College of Surgeons to the Subcommittee on Health of the Committee on Ways and Means. U.S. House of Representatives (24 May).

Baldwin, M. F. 1985. "Lawmakers Focus on Hospital-DRG Squeeze." *Modern Healthcare*. (29 March): 54–58.

Barber-Madden, R., and J. B. Kotch. 1990. "Maternity Care Financing: Universal Access or Universal Care?" *Journal of Health Politics, Policy and Law* 15 (Winter): 797–814.

Barrilleaux, C. J., and M. E. Miller. 1988. "The Political Economy of State Medicaid Policy." *The American Political Science Review* 82 (December): 1089–1108.

Bayer, R., D. Callahan, A. L. Caplan, and B. Jennings. 1988. "Toward Justice in Health Care." *American Journal of Public Health* 78: 583–88.

Beeson, P. G., and D. R. Johnson. 1987. "A Panel Study of Change (1981–1986) in Rural Mental Health Status: Effects of the Rural Crisis." Paper presented at the NIMH National Conference on Mental Health Statistics, Denver, Colorado.

Bishop, C. E. 1988. "Competition in the Market for Nursing Home Care." *The Journal of Health Politics, Policy and Law* 13 (Summer): 341–60.

Bjovberg, R. R. 1986. "Insuring the Uninsured through Private Action: Ideas and Initiatives." *Inquiry* 23: 403–18.

Blankenau, J., T. Holder, and K. J. Mueller. 1991. "A Profile of the Uninsured in Nebraska, 1990." *Quarterly Report*, vol. 1., no. 2. Omaha, Nebraska: Center for Health Services Research.

Blazer, D., L. K. George, R. Landerman, M. Pennybacker, M. L. Melville, M. Woodbury, K. G. Manton, K. Jordan, and B. Z. Locke. 1985. "Psychiatric Disorders: A Rural/Urban Comparison." *Archives of General Psychiatry* 42(no.7): 653–56.

Blendon, R. J., and J. N. Edwards. 1991. "Conclusion and Forecast for the Future." Ch.12 in R. Blendon and J. Edwards, eds." *System in Crisis: The Case for Health Care Reform*. Washington, D.C.: Faulkner & Gray.

Blendon, R. J., R. Leitman, I. Morrison., and K. Donelan. 1990. "Satisfaction with Health Systems in Ten Nations." *Health Affairs* 9 (Summer): 185–92.

Blumstein, J. F. 1989. "Government's Role in Organ Transplantation Policy." *Journal of Health Politics, Policy and Law* 14 (Spring): 5–40.

Braveman, P., G. Oliva, M. G. Miller, R. Reiter, and S. Egerter. 1989. "Adverse Outcomes and Lack of Health Insurance among Newborns in an Eight-County Area of California 1982 to 1986." *The New England Journal of Medicine* 321 (25 August): 508–13.

Braveman, P., G. Oliva, M. G. Miller, V. M. Schaaf., and R. Reiter 1988. "Women without Health Insurance: Links between Access, Poverty, Ethnicity, and Health." *Western Journal of Medicine* 149 (December): 708–11.

Breslow, L. 1990. "A Health Promotion Primer for the 1990s." *Health Affairs* 9 (Summer): 6–21.

Brightbill, T. 1991a. "Linkage Fuss Envelops Tort Reform, Medicare." *HealthWeek* 5 (25 February): 11.

———. 1991b. "Jury Still Out on Tort Reform as Malpractice Fix." *HealthWeek* 5 (11 February): 1, 31–32.

Brody, J. A. 1988. "Aging in the 20th and 21st Century." Testimony before the Joint Economic Committee, Congress of the United States. 14 June.

Brown, L. D. 1983. "Competition and Health Care Policy: Experiences and Expectations." *The Annals* 468 (July): 48–59.

———. 1988. *Health Policy in the United States: Issues and Options.* New York: Ford Foundation Occasional Paper 4.

———. 1990. "The New Activism: Federal Health Politics Revisited." *Bulletin of the New York Academy of Medicine* 66 (July–August): 293–318.

———. 1991. "The National Politics of Oregon's Rationing Plan." *Health Affairs* 10 (Summer): 28–51.

Bureau of Data Management and Strategy. 1988. *HCFA Statistics.* Washington, D.C.: U.S. Government Office. HCFA Pub. No. 03271.

Callahan, D. 1990. "Rationing Medical Progress: The Way to Affordable Health Care." *The New England Journal of Medicine* 322 (21 June): 1810–13.

Cantor, J. E. 1982. Political Action Committees: Their Evolution and Growth and Their Implications for the Political System. Washington, D.C.: Library of Congress Congressional Research Service Report No. 82-92, 6 November 1981, updated 7 May 1982.

Cassel, C. K., M. A. Rudberg, and S. J. Olshansky. 1992. "The Price of Success: Health Care in an Aging Society." *Health Affairs* 11 (Summer): 87–99.

Chassin, M. R., R. H. Brook, R. E. Park, J. Keesey, A. Fink, J. Kosecoff, K. Kahn, N. Merrick, and D. H. Solomon. 1986. "Variations in the Use of Medical and Surgical Services by the Medicare Population." *The New England Journal of Medicine* 314 (30 January): 385–90.

Checkoway, B. 1981. *Citizens and Health Care: Participation and Planning for Social Change.* New York: Pergamon Press.

Christianson, J. B., I. S. Moscovice, J. Johnson, J. Kralewski, and C. Grogan. 1990. "Evaluating Rural Hospital Consortia." *Health Affairs* 9 (Spring): 135–61.

Clausen, A. R. 1975. *How Congressmen Decide: A Policy Focus.* New York: St. Martin's Press.

Cohen, M. A., N. Kuman, and S. S. Wallack. 1992. "Who Buys Long-Term Care Insurance?" *Health Affairs* 11 (Spring): 208–23.

Colburn, D. 1985. "Physician, Organize Thyself." *Washington Post* national weekly edition (12 August): 8.

———. 1988. "As Massachusetts Goes, So Goes the Nation?" *Washington Post,* 26 April, health section.

Committee on Health Planning Goals and Standards. 1981. *Health Planning in the United States: Selected Policy Issues.* Vol. 1. Washington, D.C.: National Academy Press.

Cooper, S. K. 1990. "Curtailing Medigap Abuses the Goal of 2 Bills." *HealthWeek* 4 (26 March): 13.

———. 1991. "Health Bills Face Arduous Rite of Passage." *HealthWeek* 5 (14 January): 11–3.

Cowan, C. A., S. W. Letsch, K. R. Levit, B. T. Maple., and M. W. Stewart. 1991. "Health Care Indicators." *Health Care Financing Review* 12, no.2 (Spring): 121–40.

Cromwell, J., J. B. Mitchell, M. L. Rosenbach, W. B. Stason, and S. Hurdle. 1989. "Using Physician Time and Complexity to Identify Mispriced Procedures." *Inquiry* 26 (Spring): 7–23.

Crozier, D. A. 1984. "National Medical Care Spending." *Health Affairs* 3 (Fall): 108–20.

Cunningham, P. J., and A. C. Monheit. 1990. "Insuring the Children: A Decade of Change." *Health Affairs* 9 (Winter): 76–90.

Daniels, M. R., and J. L. Regens. 1981–82. "Physicians Assistants as a Health Care Delivery Mechanism: Incidence and Correlates of State Authorization." *Policy Studies Journal.* Special Issue: 252–60.

Daniels, N. 1985. *Just Health Care.* Cambridge: Cambridge University Press.

Davis, K. 1982. "Regulation of Hospital Costs: The Evidence on Performance." In *Financing Health Care: Competition Versus Regulation,* edited by D. Yaggy and W. G. Anlyn, 37–67. Cambridge, Mass.: Ballinger Publishing Co.

———. 1987. "Improving Access to Health Care and Assuring Catastrophic Protection for Children." Testimony before the Subcommittee on Health of the Senate Finance Committee, U.S. Congress. 2 October.

deLissovoy, G., T. Rise, J. Gabel, and H. J. Selzer. 1987. "PPOs One Year Later," *Inquiry* 24 (Summer): 127–35.

Demkovich, L. 1983. "Hospitals' Building and Buying Binge Tied to Cuts in Federal Planning Aid." *National Journal* (23 April): 832–36.

————. 1987. "The Nurse Shortage: Supply and Demand, Pay and Power." *Focus on . . .* Series No.17. Washington, D.C.: Intergovernmental Health Policy Project. August.

Derthick, M., and P. Quirk. 1985. *The Politics of Deregulation*. Washington, D.C.: The Brookings Institution.

Desharnais, S., E. Kobrinski, J. Chesney, M. Long, R. Ament, and S. Fleming. 1987. "The Early Effects of the Prospective Payment System on Inpatient Utilization and the Quality of Care." *Inquiry* 24 (Spring): 7–16.

Detroit Free Press. 1990. "Surgical Logjam Sends Canadians across Border." *Omaha World Herald* (25 February): 22A.

Diebold, J. 1984. *Making the Future Work: Unleashing Our Powers of Innovation for the Decades Ahead*. New York: Simon & Schuster.

Division of National Costs Estimates, Office of Actuary, Health Care Financing Administration. 1987. "National Health Expenditures 1986–2000." *Health Care Financing Review* 8 (Summer): 1–36.

Donham, C. S., S. W. Letsch, B. T. Maple, N. Singer, and C. A. Cowan 1991. "Health Care Indicators: Community Hospital Statistics." *Health Care Financing Review* 12 (Summer): 141–70.

Eastaugh, S. R. 1987. *Financing Health Care: Economic Efficiency and Equity*. Dover, Mass.: Auburn House.

Eckstein, H. 1960. *Pressure Group Politics: The Case of the British Medical Association*. London: Rukin House.

Ermann, D. A. 1990. "Rural Health Care: The Future of the Hospital." *Medical Care Review* 47 (Spring): 34–73.

Ermann, D., and J. Gabel. 1984. "Multihospital Systems: Issues and Empirical Findings." *Health Affairs* 3 (Spring): 50–64.

Estes, C. L. 1979. *The Aging Enterprise*. San Francisco: Jossey-Bass Publishers.

Etheredge, L., and D. Juba. 1984. "Medicare Payment for Physicians' Services." *Health Affairs* 3 (Winter): 132–37.

Evans, R. G. 1990. "Tension, Compression, and Shear: Directions, Stresses, and Outcomes of Health Care Cost Control." *Journal of Health Politics, Policy and Law* 15 (Spring): 101–28.

Evans, R. G., J. Lomas, M. L. Barber, R. J. Labelle, C. Fooks, G. L. Stoddard, G. M. Anderson, D. Feeny, A. Gafni, G. W. Torrance, and W. G. Tholl. 1986. "Cost-Effectiveness Analysis of Transplantation." *Surgical Clinics of North America* 66 (June): 603–16.

———. 1989. "Controlling Health Expenditures—The Canadian Reality." *The New England Journal of Medicine* 320 (2 March): 571–77.

Fackelmann, K. A. 1988. "Challenges Ahead for Organ Transplants." *Medicine & Health* 42 (25 January): Perspectives Insert.

Falcone, D., and L. C. Hartwig. 1991. "Congressional Process and Health Policy: Reform and Retrenchment." In *Health Politics and Policy,* 2d ed., edited by T. Litman and L. Robins, 126–44. New York: John Wiley & Sons.

Families USA Foundation. 1992. *The Health Cost Squeeze on Older Americans.* Washington, D.C.: Families USA Foundation.

Fan, D. P., and L. Norem. 1992. "The Media and the Fate of the Medicare Catastrophic Extension." *Journal of Health Politics, Policy and Law* 17 (Spring): 39–70.

Farley-Short, P., P. Kemper, L. J. Cornelius, and D. C. Walden. 1992. "Public and Private Responsibility for Financing Nursing-Home Care: The Effect of Medicaid Asset Spend-Down." *The Milbank Quarterly* 70 (no.2): 277–98.

Feder, J., J. Hadley, and S. Zuckerman. 1987. "How Did Medicare's Prospective Payment System Affect Hospitals?" *The New England Journal of Medicine* 317 (1 October): 867–73.

Feldstein, P. J. 1977. *Health Associations and the Demand for Legislation: The Political Economy of Health.* Cambridge, Mass.: Ballinger Publishing Co.

———. 1984. "Health Associations and the Legislative Process." In *Health Politics and Policy,* edited by T. Litman and L. Robins, 169–93. New York: John Wiley & Sons.

Feldstein, P. J., and G. Melnick. 1984. "Congressional Voting Behavior on Hospital Legislation: An Exploratory Study." *Journal of Health Politics, Policy and Law* 8 (Winter): 685–701.

Fiorini, M. P. 1974. *Representatives, Roll Calls, and Constituencies.* Lexington, Mass.: Lexington Books.

Firshein, J. 1990. "Is American Health Care Ripe for Reform?" *Medicine & Health* 44 (29 January): Perspectives Insert.

Fitzgerald, J. F., P. S. Moore, and R. S. Dittus. 1988. "The Care of Elderly Patients with Hip Fracture: Changes since Implementation of the Prospective Payment System." *The New England Journal of Medicine* 319 (24 November): 1392–97.

Foley, J. D. 1991. *Uninsured in the United States: The Nonelderly Population without Health Insurance.* Washington, D.C.: The Employee Benefits Research Institute.

Fossett, J. W., J. D. Perloff, P. R. Kletke, and J. A. Peterson. 1992. "Medicaid and Access to Child Health Care in Chicago." *Journal of Health Politics, Policy and Law* 17 (Summer): 273–98.

Fowler, E. M. 1987. "Nation's Nursing Shortage." *New York Times,* 1 December.

Fox, H. W., and S. W. Hammond. 1977. *Congressional Staffs: The Invisible Force in American Lawmaking.* New York: The Free Press.

Freeman, H. E., L. H. Aiken, R. J. Blendon, and C. R. Corey. 1990. "Uninsured Working-Age Adults: Characteristics and Consequences." *Health Services Research* 24 (February): 811–23.

Gaus, C., and F. Hellinger. 1976. "Results of Prospective Reimbursment." *Topics in Health Care Financing* 3 (Winter): 83–96.

General Accounting Office, GAO. 1989. "Health Insurance: An Overview of the Working Uninsured." Report to the Committee on Finance, U.S. Senate. GAO/HRD-89-45. February.

———. 1990. "Health Insurance: A Profile of the Uninsured in Michigan and the United States." Report to the Chairman, Subcommittee on Health for Families and the Uninsured, Committee on Finance, U.S. Senate. GAO/HRD-90-97. May.

Ginzberg, E. 1990. "Health Care Reform—Why So Slow?" *The New England Journal of Medicine* 322 (17 May): 1464–67.

Gonzales, M. L. 1989. "Trends, Variations, and the Distribution of Physician Earnings 1977–1988." In *Socioeconomic Characteristics of Medical Practice 1988,* edited by M. L. Gonzales and D. W. Emmons. Chicago: American Medical Association.

Gould, J. B., B. Davey, and R. S. Stafford. 1989. "Socioeconomic Differences in Rates of Cesarean Section." *The New England Journal of Medicine* 321 (27 July): 233–39.

Gray, B. H., and W. J. McNerney. 1986. "For-Profit Enterprise in Health Care: The Institute of Medicine Study." *The New England Journal of Medicine* 314 (5 June): 1523–28.

Gray, J. 1989. "How Serious Are Employers about Cutting Health Costs?" *Medical Economics* (16 October): 112–24.

Grogan, C. M. 1992. "Deciding on Access and Levels of Care: A Comparison of Canada, Britain, Germany, and the United States." *Journal of Health Politics, Policy and Law* 17 (Summer): 213–32.

Gruber, L. R., M. Shadle, and C.L. Polich. 1988. "From Movement to Industry: The Growth of HMOs." *Health Affairs* 7 (Summer): 197–208.

Guterman, S., S. H. Altman, and D. A. Young. 1990. "Hospitals' Financial Performance in the First Five Years of PPS." *Health Affairs* 9, 125–34.

Hadley, J., and K. Shwarz. 1989. "The Impacts on Hospital Costs Between 1980 and 1984 of Hospital Rate Regulation, Competition, and Changes in Health Insurance Coverage." *Inquiry* 26 (Spring): 35–47.

Hadley, J., S. Zuckerman, and J. Feder. 1989. "Profits and Fiscal Pressure in the Prospective Payment System: Their Impacts on Hospitals." *Inquiry* 16: 354–65.

Hanft, R. S. 1987. "The Need for More Physicians." *Health Affairs* 6 (Summer): 69–71.

Harnett, R. 1990. "Eight States Will Test Long-Term Care Programs." *HealthWeek* (26 March): 36.

Hart, L. G., R. A. Rosenblatt, and B. A. Amundson. 1989. "Is There a Role for the Rural Hospital?" Working Paper Series 1 (no. 1). January. University of Washington, Seattle: WAMI Rural Health Research Center.

Hart, J. P. 1988. "Rural Healthcare in Transition: A Time for Change Management." *Health Progress* (September): 31–41.

HealthWeek Staff. 1991. "HMO Market at a Glance." *HealthWeek* 5 (17 June): 24.

Hearings before the Subcommittee on Health and Scientific Research, 1979. Legislative Hearing on S. 544. 16 March.

Heclo, H. 1978. "Issue Networks and the Executive Establishment" In *The New American Political System,* edited by A. King, 87–124. Washington, D.C.: American Enterprise Institute.

Heinrich, J. 1985. "Non-Physician Providers." In *A Health Care Agenda for the States,* edited by L. Arnheim and L. Webb, 73–77. Washington, D.C.: The Conference on Alternative State and Local Policies.

Hellinger, F. J. 1991. "Forecasting the Medical Care Costs of the HIV Epidemic: 1991–1994." *Inquiry* 28 (Fall): 213–25.

Helms, W. D., A. K. Gauthier, and D. M. Campion. 1992. "Mending the Flaws in the Small-Group Market." *Health Affairs* 11 (Spring): 7–21.

Hodgson, T. A. 1992. "Cigarette Smoking and Lifetime Medical Expenditures." *The Milbank Quarterly* 70 (no. 1): 81–126.

Holahan, J., and S. Zedlewski. 1991. "Expanding Medicaid to Cover Uninsured Americans." *Health Affairs* 10 (Spring): 45–61.

Holden, K. C., and T. M. Smeeding. 1990. "The Poor, the Rich, and the Insecure Elderly Caught in Between." *The Milbank Quarterly* 68 (no. 2): 191–220.

Horowitz, M. G. 1988. "Montana Grapples with Obstetrics Crisis in Rural Areas." *HealthWeek* (1 February): 16.

Hosenball, M. 1989. "And Seal It With a Hiss." *Washington Post* national weekly edition (30 October–5 November): 24.

House of Representatives. 1989. *Omnibus Reconciliation Act of 1989: Conference Report to Accompany H.R. 3299.* Washington, D.C.: U.S. Government Printing Office. 21 November.

Howell, J. R. 1984. "Evaluating the Impact of Certificate-of-Need Regulation Using Measures of Ultimate Outcome: Some Cautions from Experience in Massachusetts." *Health Services Research* 19, no.5 (December): 587–613.

Hsiao, W. C., P. Braun, D. Yntema, and E. R. Becker. 1988. "Estimating Physicians' Work for a Resource-Based Relative-Value Scale." *The New England Journal of Medicine,* 319: 835–41.

Hughes, D., and S. Rosenbaum. 1989. "An Overview of Maternal and Infant Health Services in Rural America." *The Journal of Rural Health* 5 (October): 299–320.

Hudson, E. 1988. "Texas Leads Fight to Halt 'Patient-Dumping' by Private Hospitals." *Washington Post* (20 March): A4.

Iglehart, J. K. 1975a. "Health Report/Congress Expands Capacity to Contest Executive Policy." *National Journal Reports* (17 May): 730–39.

———. 1975b. "Health Report/State, County Governments Win Key Roles in New Program." *National Journal* (8 November): 1533–39.

———. 1982a. "New Jersey's Experiment with DRG-Based Hospital Reimbursement." *The New England Journal of Medicine* 307: 1655–60.

———. 1982b. "The New Era of Prospective Payment for Hospitals." *The New England Journal of Medicine,* 307: 1288–92.

———. 1985. "The Administration's Assault on Domestic Spending and the Threat to Health Care Programs." *The New England Journal of Medicine* 312 (21 February): 525–28.

———. 1986. "Early Experience with Prospective Payment of Hospitals." *The New England Journal of Medicine* 314 (29 May): 1460–64.

———. 1989a. "Medicare's New Benefits: 'Catastrophic' Health Insurance." *The New England Journal of Medicine* 320 (2 February): 329–35.

———. 1989b. "The Recommendations of the Physician Payment Review Commission." *The New England Journal of Medicine* 320: 1156–60.

———. 1990. "Canada's Health Care System Faces Its Problems." *The New England Journal of Medicine* 322 (22 February): 562–68.

Interstudy. 1989. "The InterStudy Edge, 1989," vol.4. *Medical Benefits* 7 (15 January): 3–4.

Jacobsen, S. J., and A. A. Rimm. 1987. "The Projected Physician Surplus Reevaluated." *Health Affairs* 6 (Summer): 48–56.

Jones, R., and P. Woll. 1979. *The Private World of Congress.* New York: The Free Press.

Jonsen, A. R. 1990. *The New Medicine and the Old Ethics.* Cambridge, Mass.: Harvard University Press.

Karpatkin, R. H. 1991. "Hearing before the Subcommittee on Health." *Committee on Finance* (16 April): 103–13.

Kasper, J. D. 1988. *Aging Alone: Profiles and Projections.* A Report of the Commonwealth Fund Commission on Elderly People Living Alone. Baltimore, Md.

Kass, N. E., R. R. Faden, R. Fox, and J. Dudley. 1991. "Loss of Private Health Insurance Among Homosexual Men with AIDS." *Inquiry* 28 (Fall): 249–54.

Kelman, S. 1987. "Public Choice and Public Spirit." *The Public Interest* 87 (Spring): 80–94.

Kimball, M. C. 1990. "Nation's Health Bill To Rise 10.4% in 1990, U.S. Says." *HealthWeek* 4, no. 1 (8 January): 1, 52.

Kingdon, J. 1984. *Agendas, Alternatives, and Public Policies.* Boston: Little, Brown.

———. 1988. Ideas, Politics, and Public Policies. Paper presented at the 1988 Annual Meeting of the American Political Association.

Kirkman-Liff, B. L. 1990. "Physician Payment and Cost-Containment Strategies in West Germany: Suggestions for Medicare Reform." *Journal of Health Politics, Policy and Law* 15 (Spring): 69–100.

Koitz, D., J. Reuter, and M. Merlis. 1989. "Medicare: Its Use, Funding, and Economic Dimensions." Prepared at the Request of the U.S. Senate Committee on Finance. 1 March.

Kosterlitz, J. 1986. "Picking Up the Tab." *National Journal* (26 July): 1825–28.

———. 1989a. "But Not for Us?" *National Journal* (22 July): 1871–75.

———. 1989b. "Taking Care of Canada." *National Journal* (15 July): 1792–97.

Kralewski, J. E., B. Dowd, R. Feldman, and J. Shapiro. 1987. "The Physician Rebellion." *The New England Journal of Medicine* 316 (5 February): 339–42.

Lazenby, H. C., and S. W. Letsch. 1990. "National Health Expenditures 1989." *Health Care Financing Review* 12 (Winter): 1–26.

Leberto, T. 1988. "Top 25 Investor-Owned Hospital Management Companies." *HealthWeek* (1 February): 32.

Lee, P. R., and C. L. Estes. 1983. "New Federalism and Health Policy." *The Annals of the American Academy of Political and Social Science* 468: 88–102.

Lemov, P. 1990. "Health Insurance For All: A Possible Dream?" *Governing* (November): 56–62.

Letsch, S. W., K. R. Levit, and D. R. Waldo. 1988. "National Health Expenditures 1987." *Health Care Financing Review* 10 (Winter): 109–29.

Levine, P. B. 1984. "An Overview of the State Role in the United States Health Scene." In *Health Politics and Policy,* edited by T. Litman and L. Robins, 194–220. New York: John Wiley & Sons.

Levit, K. R., and C. A. Cowan. 1991. "Business, Households, and Governments: Health Care Costs, 1990." *Health Care Financing Review* 11 (Winter): 83–93.

Levit, K. R., and M. S. Freeland. 1988. "National Medical Care Spending." *Health Affairs* 7. (Winter): 124–36.

Levit, K. R., H. C. Lazenby, C. A. Cowan, and S. W. Letsch. 1991. "National Health Expenditures, 1990." *Health Care Financing Review* 13 (Fall): 29–54.

Lieberman, M. 1987. "Physicians' Discipline in New York State: Political and Policy Issues." Paper delivered at the 1987 Annual Meeting of the American Political Science Association. Chicago, Ill.

Lindblom, C. E. 1965. *The Intelligence of Democracy.* New York: The Free Press.

———. 1979. "Still Muddling: Not Yet Through." *Public Administration Review* 39 (November/December): 417–26.

Lister, J. 1986. "The Politics of Medicine in Britain and the United States." Shattuck Lecture. *The New England Journal of Medicine* 315 (17 July): 168–73.

Litman, T., and L. Robins. 1991. *Health Politics and Policy.* 2d ed. New York: John Wiley & Sons.

Long, S. H. 1985. "Medicare Reform: What Are the Options?" In *Medicare Reform: The Private-Sector Impact,* 1–6. Washington, D.C.: Employee Benefit Research Institute.

Lurie, N., N. B. Ward, M. F. Shapiro, C. Gallego, R. Vaghaiwalla, and R. H. Brook. 1986. "Termination of Medi-Cal Benefits: A Follow-up Study One Year Later." *The New England Journal of Medicine* 314 (8 May): 1266–68.

McCloskey, A. H., and J. Luehrs. 1990. *State Initiatives to Improve Rural Health Care.* Washington D.C.: National Governor's Association.

McEachern, S. 1990. "Colorado May Ration Health Care." *HealthWeek* (7 May): 8.

McKinlay, J. B., and J. Arches. 1985. "Towards the Proletarianization of Physicians." *International Journal of Health Services* 15 (2): 161–95.

Malbin, M. J. 1980. *Unelected Representatives: Congressional Staff and the Future of Representative Government.* New York: Basic Books.

Managed Health Care. 1989. (4 December): 1, 11.

Manning, W. G., A. Leibowitz, G. A. Goldberg, W. H. Rogers, and J. P. Newhouse. 1984. "A Controlled Trial of the Effect of a Prepaid Group Practice on Use of Services." *The New England Journal of Medicine* 310 (7 June): 1505–10.

Marder, W. D., D. W. Emmons, P. R. Kletke, and R. J. Wilke. 1988. "Physician Employment Patterns." *Health Affairs* 7 (Winter): 137–45.

Marion Laboratories. 1989. Marion Managed Care Digest PPO Edition—1989. *Medical Benefits* 7 (15 January): 1–2.

Marmor, T. 1973. *The Politics of Medicare*. Chicago: Aldine Publishing Co.

Marmor, T. R., and J. B. Christianson. 1982. *Health Care Policy: A Political Economy Approach*. Beverly Hills: Sage.

Mayer, D., and M. C. Kimball. 1991. "Ore. Commission OKs Medicaid Pecking Order." *HealthWeek* 5 (no.1): 36.

Medicine & Health. 1990. (15 January): 1.

———. 1992. Vol.46, no.1 (16 March): 2.

Mick, S. S., and L. L. Morlock. 1990. "America's Rural Hospitals: A Selective Review of 1980s Research." *The Journal of Rural Health* 6 (October): 437–66.

Minor, A. F. 1989. "The Cost of Maternity Care and Childbirth in the United States, 1989." *Research Bulletin* December R1589. Washington, D.C.: Health Insurance Association of America.

Morone, J. A. 1990a. *The Democratic Wish: Popular Participation and the Limits of American Government*. New York: Basic Books.

———. 1990b. "Beyond the Words: The Politics of Health Care Reform." *Bulletin of the New York Academy of Medicine* 66: 344–65.

———. 1990c. "American Political Culture and the Search for Lessons from Abroad." *Journal of Health Politics, Policy and Law* 15 (Spring): 129–44.

Mueller, K. J. 1984. "Local Government Implementation of Nationally Inspired Programs: A Comparative Analysis." *Journal of Urban Affairs* 6 (Spring): 166–78.

———. 1985. "The Development of Health Policy in the U.S. Congress." Paper delivered at the 1985 Annual Meeting of the American Political Science Association, Washington, D.C.

———. 1986. "An Analysis of Congressional Health Policy Voting in the 1970s." *Journal of Health Politics, Policy and Law* 11 (Spring): 117–35.

———. 1988a. "Federal Programs Do Expire: The Case of Health Planning." *Public Administration Review* 48 (May/June): 719–25.

———. 1988b. "The Role of Policy Analysis in Agenda Setting: Applications to the Problem of Indigent Health Care in the United States." *Policy Studies Journal* 16 (Spring): 441–53.

———. 1988c. "State Regulation of Rural Hospitals: Innovations in the 1980s." *Focus On . . .* Series. Washington, D.C.: The Intergovernmental Health Policy Project. October.

———. 1989. "The National Organ Transplant Act of 1984: Congressional Response to Changing Biotechnology." *Policy Studies Review* 8 (Winter): 346–56.

Mueller, K. J., and J. C. Comer. 1983. "Dissinovation in the American States: Policy toward Health System Agencies." *Journal of Sociology and Social Welfare* 10 (June): 189–202.

———. 1991. "The Case of Health Systems Agencies: Some Correlates of Health Policy in the States." *State and Local Government Review* 23 (Winter): 13–16.

Mullen, P. 1991. "Mass. Loses Its Faith in Miracles: The Universal Health Care Bubble Bursts." *HealthWeek* 5, no. 1: 33–34.

Mundinger, M. O. 1985. "Health Service Funding Cuts and the Declining Health of the Poor." *The New England Journal of Medicine* 313 (4 July): 44–47.

Munts, R. 1967. *Bargaining for Health: Labor Unions, Health Insurance, and Medical Care.* Madison: University of Wisconsin Press.

Murray, J. D., and P. A. Keller. 1991. "Psychology and Rural America: Current Status and Future Directions." *American Psychologist* 46 (March): 220–31.

Mushlin, A. I., R. J. Panzer, E. R. Black, P. Greenland, and D. I. Regenstreif. 1988. "Quality of Care During a Community-wide Experiment in Prospective Payment to Hospitals." *Medical Care* 26 (November): 1081–91.

Myers, S. A., and N. Gleicher. 1988. "A Successful Program to Lower Cesarean-Section Rates." *The New England Journal of Medicine* 319 (8 December): 1511–16.

National Commission on Acquired Immune Deficiency Syndrome. 1991. *America Living with AIDS.* Washington, D.C.: National Commission on Acquired Immune Deficiency Syndrome.

Naylor, C. D. 1986. *Private Practice, Public Payment: Canadian Medicine and the Politics of Health Insurance, 1911–1966.* Kingston: McGill-Queen's University Press.

Neighbors, H. W., and J. S. Jackson. 1987. "Barriers to Medical Care among Adult Blacks: What Happens to the Uninsured?" *Journal of the National Medical Association* 79 (no.5): 489–93.

New York Times. 1988. "Florida Special Session to Weigh Crisis Over Physicians' Insurance." (2 February): A 19.

New York Times. 1991. "Canada Runs Out of Money for Health Care." Reprinted in *Omaha World Herald* (8 December): B-2.

Newhouse, J. P., G. Anderson, and L. L. Roos. 1988. "Hospital Spending in the United States and Canada." *Health Affairs* 7 (Winter): 6–16.

Oberg, C. N. 1990. "Medically Uninsured Children in the United States: A Challenge to Public Policy." *Pediatrics* 85: 824–32.

O'Connor, K. 1990. "Program for Uninsured in Wash. Slowly Growing." *HealthWeek* 4: 40–41.

Office of Disease Prevention and Health Promotion. 1988. *Disease Prevention/Health*

Promotion. Washington, D.C.: U.S. Public Health Service, U.S. Department of Health and Human Services.

Office of Technology Assessment, OTA. 1990. *Health Care in Rural America*. Washington, D.C.: U.S. Government Printing Office.

O'Sullivan, J. 1988. *Medicare: Physician Payments*. Issue Brief IB/85-007. Washington, D.C.: Congressional Research Service.

Patton, L. T. 1988. "The Rural Health Care Challenge." Staff Report to the Special Committee On Aging, U.S. Senate. October. Washington, D.C.: U.S. Government Printing Office.

Pawlson, L. G. 1988. "The Future of Health Care in America: Current and Projected Health Status of the Elderly." Testimony before the Joint Economic Committee, Congress of the United States. 14 June.

Pear, R. 1988. "Expanded Right to Medicaid Shatters the Link to Welfare." *New York Times* (6 March): 1.

Pepper Commission Report. 1990. *Health Care for All Americans*. Washington, D.C.: U.S. Government Printing Office.

Perrin, J. M., C. J. Homer, D. M. Berwick, A. D. Woolf, J. L. Freeman, and J. E. Wennberg. 1989. "Variations in Rates of Hospitalization of Children in Three Urban Counties." *The New England Journal of Medicine* 320 (4 May): 1183–87.

Piper, J. M., W. A. Ray, and M. R. Griffin. 1990. "Effects of Medicaid Eligibilty Expansion on Prenatal Care and Pregnancy Outcome in Tennessee." *Journal of the American Medical Association* 264 (7 November): 2219–23.

Pfaff, M. 1990. "Differences in Health Care Spending Across Countries: Statistical Evidence." *Journal of Health Politics, Policy and Law* 15 (Spring): 1–68.

Quirk, P. 1988. "In Defense of the Politics of Ideas." *The Journal of Politics* 50 (February): 31–41.

Reagan, M. D. 1987. "Physicians as Gatekeepers: A Complex Challenge." *The New England Journal of Medicine* 317 (31 December): 1731–34.

Relman, A. S. 1980. "The New Medical-Industrial Complex." *The New England Journal of Medicine* 303 (23 October): 963–70.

Rich, S. 1990. "The Working Poor: Lost in a Health Care No-Man's Land." *Washington Post* (18–24 June): 7.

Ries P. 1991. "Characteristics of Persons with and without Health Care Coverage: United States, 1989." Advance Data No.201. "Washington, D.C.: National Center for Health Statistics. 18 June.

Riffer, J. 1985. "Home Care Agencies Up 25 Percent Since '84." *Hospitals* (16 May): 64–65.

Ripley, R. 1972. *The Politics of Economic and Human Resource Development*. Indianapolis: The Bobbs-Merrill Co.

Robach, G., L. Randolph, B. Seidman, and D. Mead. 1992. *1992 Edition Physician Characteristics and Distribution in the United States*. Chicago: The American Medical Association.

Robert Wood Johnson Foundation. 1987. "Access to Health Care in the United States: Results of a 1986 Survey." *Special Report*. Princeton, N.J.: Robert Wood Johnson Foundation.

Roe, B. B. 1981. "The UCR Boondoggle: A Death Knell for Private Practice?" *The New England Journal of Medicine* 305: 41–45.

Roper, W. L. 1988. "Perspectives on Physician-Payment Reform." *The New England Journal of Medicine* 319: 865–68.

Roper, W. L., and G. M. Hackbarth. 1988. HCFA's Agenda for Promoting High-Quality Care." *Health Affairs* 7 (Spring): 91–98.

Rosenbach, M. L., and A. G. Stone. 1990. "Malpractice Insurance Costs." *Health Affairs* 9 (Winter): 176–85.

Rosenbaum, S., D. D. Hughes, and K. Johnson 1988. "Maternal and Child Health Services for Medically Indigent Children and Pregnant Women." *Medical Care* 26 (April): 315–32.

Rosenblatt, R. A, and I. S. Moscovice. 1982. *Rural Health Care*. New York: John Wiley & Sons.

Rosenberg, C. E. 1979. "Inward Vision and Outward Glance: The Shaping of the American Hospital, 1880–1914." *Bulletin of the History of Medicine* 53: 346–91.

Rosko, M. D. 1984. "The Impact of Prospective Payment: A Multi-Dimensional Analysis of New Jersey's SHARE Program." *Journal of Health Politics, Policy and Law* 79: 81–102.

Rostow, V. P., M. Osterweis, and R. J. Bulger. 1989. "Medical Professional Liability and the Delivery of Obstetrical Care." *The New England Journal of Medicine* 321 (12 October): 1057–60.

Rowland, D., and B. Lyons. 1987. *Medicare's Poor: Filling the Gaps in Medical Coverage for Low-Income Elderly Americans*. Baltimore: The Commonwealth Fund Commission on Elderly People Living Alone.

Rovner, J. 1990. "No Help From Congress on a Near-Term Solution For Long-Term Care." *Governing* (June): 21–27.

———. 1989. "Repeal of Medicare Law Brings Back Old Limits." *Congressional Quarterly* (2 December): 3330–31.

Russell, L. B., and C. L. Manning. 1989. "The Effect of Prospective Payment on Medicare Expenditures." *The New England Journal of Medicine* 320 (16 February): 439–44.

St. Peter, R. F., P. W. Newacheck, and N. Halfon. 1992. "Access to Care for Poor Children: Separate and Unequal?" *Journal of the American Medical Association* 267 (27 May): 2760–64.

Salamon, L. M., and J. J. Siegfried. 1977. "Economic Power and Political Influence: The Impact of Industry Structure on Public Policy." *The American Political Science Review* 71 (September): 1026–43.

Salkever, D. S., and T. W. Bice. 1976. "The Impact of Certificate-of-Need Controls on Hospital Investment." *Milbank Memorial Fund Quarterly* 54 (Spring): 195–214.

Salive, M. E., J. A. Mayfield, and N. W. Weissman. 1990. "Patient Outcomes Research Teams and the Agency for Health Care Policy and Research." *Health Services Research* 25 (December): 697–708.

Sapolsky, H. M. 1986. "Prospective Payment in Perspective." *Journal of Health Politics, Policy and Law* 11 (no.3) : 633–46.

Sardell, A. 1990. "Child Health Policy in the U.S.: The Paradox of Consensus." *Journal of Health Care Politics, Policy and Law* 15 (Summer): 271–304.

Schieber, G. J. 1990. "Health Expenditures in Major Industrialized Countries, 1960–87." *Health Care Financing Review* 11 (Summer): 159–68.

Schlesinger, M., and K. Kronebusch. 1990. "The Failure of Prenatal Care Policy for the Poor." *Health Affairs* 9 (Winter): 91–111.

Schloss, E. P. 1988. "Beyond GMENAC—Another Physician Shortage from 2010 to 2030?" *The New England Journal of Medicine* 318 (7 April): 920–22.

Schmidt, S. 1988. "Md. Moves to Punish Bad Doctors." *Washington Post* (7 April): A1.

Schneider, E. L. 1989. "Options to Control the Rising Health Care Costs of Older Americans." *Journal of the American Medical Association* 26 (February): 907–8.

Schwartz, W. B., F. A. Sloan, and D. N. Mendelson. 1988. "Why There Will Be Little or No Physician Surplus between Now and the Year 2000." *The New England Journal of Medicine* 318 (7 April): 892–97.

Short, P. F., A. Monheit, and K. Beauregard. 1988. "Uninsured Americans: A 1987 Profile." Paper presented at the Annual Meetings of the American Public Health Association in Boston, Mass., 13–18 November.

Sloan, F. A. 1988. "Property Rights in the Hospital Industry." In *Health Care in America: The Political Economy of Hospitals and Health Insurance,* edited by H. E. French III, 103–43. San Francisco: Pacific Institute for Public Policy.

Sloan, F. A., and B. Steinwald. 1980. "Effects of Regulation on Hospital Costs and Input Use." *Journal of Law and Economics* 23 (April): 81–109.

Smith, H. 1988. *The Power Game: How Washington Works.* New York: Random House.

Smith, M. D., D. E. Altman, R. Leitman, T. W. Moloney, and H. Taylor. 1992. "Taking the Public's Pulse on Health System Reform." *Health Affairs* 11 (Summer): 125–33.

Smith, R. A. 1984. "Advocacy, Interpretation, and Influence in the U.S. Congress." *The American Political Science Review* 78 (March): 44–63.

Somers, A. R. 1969. *Hospital Regulation: The Dilemma of Public Policy.* Princeton, N.J.: Industrial Relations Section, Princeton University.

Sorian, R. 1988. "Stark Proposes Planning Redux." *Medicine & Health* 42 (12 September): 1.

Southwick, K. 1990. "Ore. Blazing a Trail with Plan to Ration Health Care." *Health-Week* (12 March): 30–33

Specter, M. 1987. "Florida's Malpractice Crisis Is Closing Emergency Rooms." *Washington Post* (27 July): 32–33.

———. 1991. "Unhealthy Care for the Poor: New York Has Symptoms of Medicaid in Crisis." *Washington Post* (15–21 July): 9.

Stark, P. 1988. "Perspectives." *Health Affairs* 7 (Winter): 35–36.

Starr, P. 1982a. *The Social Transformation of American Medicine.* New York: Basic Books.

———. 1982b. "The Triumph of Accommodation: The Rise of Private Health Plans in America 1929–1959." *The Journal of Health Politics, Policy and Law* 7 (Fall): 580–628.

Stevens, C. 1989a. "Why Business Is Rushing to Support NHI." *Medical Economics* 21 (August): 132–46.

———. 1989b. "Here's What RBRVS Will Really Do to Your Income." *Medical Economics* (15 May): 19–34.

Stevens, R. 1982. " 'A Poor Sort of Memory': Voluntary Hospitals and Government before the Depression." *Milbank Memorial Fund Quarterly* 60 (Fall): 551–84.

———. 1986. "The Future of the Medical Profession." In *From Physician Shortage to Patient Shortage: The Future of Medical Practice,* edited by E. Ginzberg, 75–93. Denver: Westview Press.

Subcommittee on Health and the Environment, Committee on Energy and Commerce, U.S. House of Representatives. 1982. "Extension of the Health Planning Program Hearings." 22 March. Washington, D.C.: Government Printing Office.

Summer, L. 1991. *Limited Access: Health Care for the Rural Poor.* Washington, D.C.: Center on Budget and Policy Priorities.

Swartz, K. 1990. "Why Requiring Employers to Provide Health Insurance Is a Bad Idea." *Journal of Health Politics, Policy and Law* 15 (Winter): 779–92.

Sylvester, K. 1990. "New Jersey Reaches Out to Moms-to-Be." *Governing* (March): 12.

Tallon, J. R. 1990. "Medicaid: Challenges and Opportunities." *Health Care Financing Review* (1990 Annual Supplement): 5–8.

Taylor, H., R. Leitman, and J. N. Edwards. 1991. "Physicians' Responses to Their Changing Environment." In *System in Crisis: The Case for Health Care Reform,* edited by R. Blendon and J. Edwards, ch.7. Washington, D.C.: Faulkner and Gray.

Taylor, M. G. 1978. *Health Insurance and Canadian Public Policy: The Seven Decisions That Created the Canadian Health Insurance System.* Montreal: McGill-Queen's University Press.

Temin, P. 1988. "An Economic History of American Hospitals." In *Health Care in America,* edited by H. E. French III, 75–102. San Francisco: Pacific Research Institute for Public Policy.

Thorpe, K. E. 1988. "The Use of Regression Analysis to Determine Hospital Payment: The Case of Medicare's Indirect Teaching Adjustment." *Inquiry* 25: 219–31.

Vall-Spinosa, A. 1991. "Lessons from London: The British are Reforming Their National Health Service." *American Journal of Public Health* 81 (December): 1566–70.

Wacker, R. C., D. F. Reczynski, and B. D. Tibbs. 1987. *Environmental Assessment Overview 1987.* Chicago: The American Hospital Association.

Wagenfeld, M. O. 1990. "Mental Health and Rural America: A Decade Review." *The Journal of Rural Health* 6 (October): 507–22.

Washington Post. 1988. "Out-of-State Move Averts Discipline." (10 January): A17

Watt, J. M., R. A. Derzon, S. C. Renn, C. J. Schramm, J. S. Hahn, and G. D. Pillari. 1986. "The Comparative Economic Performance of Investor-Owned Chain and Not-For-Profit Hospitals." *The New England Journal of Medicine* 314 (9 January): 89–96.

Waxman, Hon. H. A. 1987. "Medical Malpractice and Quality of Care." *The New England Journal of Medicine* 316 (9 April): 943–44.

Weisman, C. S., L. L. Morlock, M. A. Teitelbaum, A. C. Klassen, and D. D. Celentano. 1989. "Practice Changes in Response to the Malpractice Litigation Climate." *Medical Care* 27 (January): 16–24.

Wennberg, J. 1986. "Which Rate is Right?" *The New England Journal of Medicine* 314 (30 January): 310–11.

Wennberg, J. E., K. McPherson, and P. Caper. 1984. "Will Payment Based on Diagnosis-Related Groups Control Hospital Costs?" *The New England Journal of Medicine* 311 (2 August): 295–300.

Wiener, J. O. 1991a. "Health Care Reform: It Won't Come Easy." *Medicine & Health* 45, "Perspectives."

———. 1991b. "Physician Payment Reform: Struggling to Be Born." *Medicine & Health* 45, "Perspectives."

Williams, T. F. 1988. "Statement to the U.S. Congress Joint Economic Committee." 14 June.

Wilson, B. L. 1991. "Health Insurance Plan Hopes to Ease Access." *Governing* (March): 14–15.

Witt, H. 1989. "Canada Cares for All—Eventually." *Omaha World Herald* (12 March): 20-A.

Wysong, J. A., and T. Abel. 1990. "Universal Health Insurance and High-Risk Groups in West Germany: Implications for U.S. Health Policy." *The Milbank Quarterly* 68 (no.4): 527–60.

Zuckerman, S., and J. Holahan. 1988. PPS Waivers: Implications for Medicare, Medicaid, and Commercial Insurers." *Journal of Health Politics, Policy and Law* 13: 663–82.

Index

AARP. *See* American Association of Retired Persons
AFDC. *See* Aid to Families with Dependent Children
Agency for Health Care, Policy, and Research (AHCPR), 11, 137, 144, 175
AHA. *See* American Hospital Association
AHCPR. *See* Agency for Health Care, Policy, and Research
AHPA. *See* American Health Planning Association
AIDS, 39, 133–39, 180, 182–83
Aid to Families with Dependent Children (AFDC), 107–8
Allied Health Professionals, 177–78
AMA. *See* American Medical Association
Ambulatory Surgical Centers, 46
American Association of Retired Persons (AARP), 19; Medicare Catastrophic Act and, 30
American Health Planning Association (AHPA), 70, 73
American Hospital Association (AHA), 85
American Medical Association (AMA), 5, 19, 32; national health insurance and, 31, 158

Bowmen, Otis R., 117
Brown, L. D., 167
Bush, President George, 140–41

Canada, 155
Canadian Health Care System, 159–64; cost control in, 162–64; difference between U.S. and, 160–62; problems with, 163–64; rationed care in, 162–63
Canadian Medical Association, 159
Carter, President Jimmy, 79
Certificate of Need (CON), 7, 22, 70, 75–76
Cesarean sections, 142
Childbirth, 9
Chronic health problems, 151–52
Clinton, President Bill, 173
COBRA. *See* Consolidated Omnibus Budget Reconciliation Act of 1985
CON. *See* Certificate of Need
Congressional voting behavior, 22–23; technical issues and, 24–25; variables of, 23–24
Consolidated Omnibus Budget Reconciliation Act of 1985 (COBRA), 92
Cost containment, 32, 58–60; in Canada, 162; and hospitals, 59–60; in maternity

Cost containment (*cont.*)
  care, 9; medical finance reform and,
  171–72; physicians and, 60–61; policies,
  180–82
Cost effective analysis, 2
Cyclosporine, 146–47. *See also* Technology

Deficit Reduction Act of 1984, 92
Diagnosis Related Groups (DRGS), 78, 80;
  rural hospitals and, 85; variations of,
  84–85
DRGS see Diagnosis Related Groups
Durenberger, Senator David, 28

Economically motivated decisions, 2
Elderly: access problems of, 113–20; near-
  poor, 120; needs of, 113–14; and
  supplemental insurance, 114
Environmental hazards, 150–51
Environmental Protection Agency (EPA),
  150
EPA. *See* Environmental Protection Agency

Federal deficit, 82
Feldstein, Paul, 19, 22
Flexner report, 4
For-profit hospitals, 44–46; vs. non-profit
  hospitals, 44–46

Geographic access to health care, 10
Ginzburg, E., 169
"Global Budgeting," 78
Great Britain, 155. *See also* Western
  nations; Industrialized nations
Gore, Vice President Albert, 146, 168

Hatch, Senator Orrin, 140
HCFA. *See* Health Care Finance
  Administration
Health care: affordability of, 112; as a social
  good, 2

Health care, access to: as a right, 1; and
  charity care, 5; cultural barriers and,
  106; economic barriers to, 106; of
  elderly, 6, 9–10, 113–20; expanding,
  179–80; in inner cities,132; financial
  problems and, 9–10, 100–101, 180;
  geographic, 100–101; government
  policy and, 2–3; by low-income
  individuals, 6, 131–33; Medicaid and,
  106–8; of the middle class, 6; and
  minimum level of service, 2;
  opportunities for, 107; policy
  environment and, 105; the poor and, 6;
  and private insurance, 6–7; problems
  with, 180; by rural residents, 120–31;
  states and, 110–13
Health care costs. *See* Health care
  expenditures
Health care delivery, 11–14, 42–53; access
  and, 167; competition and, 79;
  corporations, 12–13; economics of, 13;
  individual providers and, 46–53;
  institutions, 42–46
Health care expenditures, 41, 53–65, 167,
  177; complexity of, 41; cost containment and, 166–67; federal budget and,
  79; government involvement in, 54;
  health planning and, 71; hospital care
  and, 46, 58–60; increases in, 54–56,
  61–64; and individual costs, 54; in industrialized nations, 156–57; inflation
  and, 55–56; and lessons from Canada,
  161; percentage of GNP, 54–56; physician services and, 58; population
  growth and, 62; and private health
  insurance, 54; technology and, 62–63
Health care finance, 157–58; in Germany,
  157
Health Care Finance Administration
  (HCFA), 137, 143